Early Parenting and Later Child Achievement

Special Aspects of Education

A series of books edited by Roy Evans, Roehampton Institute, London, UK

This book is part of a series. The publisher will accept continuation orders which may be cancelled at any time and which provide for automatic billing and shipping of each title in the series upon publication. Please write for details.

Early Parenting and Later Child Achievement

Edited by

ALICE STERLING HONIG

Syracuse University, New York, USA

GORDON   AND   BREACH   SCIENCE   PUBLISHERS
New York Philadelphia London Paris Montreux Tokyo Melbourne

Gordon and Breach Science Publishers

Post Office Box 786
Cooper Station
New York, New York 10276
United States of America

5301 Tacony Street, Slot 330
Philadelphia, Pennsylvania 19137
United States of America

Post Office Box 197
London WC2E 9PX
United Kingdom

58, rue Lhomond
75005 Paris
France

Post Office Box 161
1820 Montreux 2
Switzerland

3-14-9, Okubo
Shinjuku-ku, Tokyo 169
Japan

Private Bag 8
Camberwell, Victoria 3124
Australia

The articles published in this book first appeared in *Early Child Development and Care*,
Volume 27, Number 2.

Library of Congress Cataloging-in-Publication Data

Early parenting and later child achievement / edited by Alice Sterling
  Honig.
      p.   cm. -- (Special aspects of education ; v. 14)
    "The articles published in this book first appeared in Early child
  development and care, volume 27" -- T.p. verso.
    Includes index.
    ISBN 2-88124-7770-9
    1. Parenting. 2. Education -- Parent participation. I. Honig,
  Alice S. II. Series.
  HQ755.8.E17   1990
  306.874--dc20
  ISSN 0731-8413   90–43998
                                                                             CIP

Contents

Introduction to the Series

Increasingly in the last 10 to 15 years the published literature within the field of care education has become more specialized and focused: an inevitable consequence of the information explosion and the wider scope of theoretical and practical knowledge being required of students in both the traditional and developing areas of professional training. Students within initial and post-initial training evidently need to have ready access to specialized theoretical and pedagogical resources relevant to the context of their future professional involvements which also develop special aspects of an area of study in a critically evaluative way.

In the study of education and pedagogy, the analytical and experimental approaches of psychology, philosophy, sociology, social anthropology etc., have provided insights into teaching and learning, into schooling and education. Historically these disciplines have focused their attention on relatively homogeneous populations. Increased worldwide mobility has created a need for a more pluralistic approach to education — particularly in Western countries — and a more broadly based concern for educational issues related in particular contexts. Hence, further literature has developed in recent years that is concerned with the pedagogical and curricular issues raised, for example, in connection with the "urban school", minority ethnic groups, disadvantaged and handicapped groups, and children who live apart from their families.

What is frequently missing from discipline-oriented studies is a real appreciation of context beyond the "general". What is often not present in the contextual study is an interdisciplinary analysis of the issue that provides a framework for practice.

The present series — "Special Aspects of Education" — is intended to bridge the gap between the problems of practice, as perceived in a variety of contexts, and theory, as derived from a variety of disciplines. Books accepted or commissioned for inclusion in the series will manifestly be expected to acknowledge the interdisciplinary nature of the issues and problems in the field of education and care, and, addressing themselves to particular contexts, to provide a conceptual framework for identifying and meeting special educational needs.

Roy Evans

Early parenting and later child achievement

INTRODUCTION

Contemporary researchers are fully aware of the multidimensionality of factors that affect children's achievement outcomes. Societal effects, peer effects, teacher influences, and the contribution of the child's *own* behaviors on parents can all shape the ultimate levels of child cognitive and academic competence and personal adjustment. More is known now also about genetic contributions—from temperament to absolute musical pitch—to child outcomes. But there is still a passionate interest in tracing the ways in which variations in early parental rearing philosophies and techniques eventuate or not in later child achievement characteristics. This interest becomes acute when the troubling statistics on high educational dropout rates for some groups of children are considered.

For decades, evidence has been available that *structural* demographic variables, such as parental education and income level, were significantly associated with child schooling success. But socio-economic variables do not account for the complexity of child achievement outcomes. More evidence has become available within the past quarter century that family *process* variables and parental expectancies, values, responsivities, and tutorial efforts are equally if not more dynamically related to children's later achievements. Indeed, presumption of causal relationship between different rearing styles and differential achievements in academic endeavors led to creative conceptualizations of early curricula for parents. In the '60s and '70s there was an intense flurry of activity to create innovative enrichment projects, many of which reached out to teach parenting skills (Honig, 1979) so that families could enhance the quality of their rearing and education efforts with their children.

The set of research reports collected here represents an exciting variety of efforts to relate earlier parental status, styles, attitudes, educational practices, and interaction patterns with infants and young children to later child achievement.

1

These longitudinal studies report use of a *variety* of methods to measure parental milieux and processes that can be facilitative of or inimical to achievements and adjustments of children. Some of these studies measure parental-child differences from the earliest days. Dr. Ringler's work looks at the long-term potential effects on language/meaning interactions between mothers and children from low income, disadvantaged families where an intervention procedure a decade earlier provided extra contact between mother and newborn infant to one group but not to the control group. Other studies in this collection did not begin data collection until the children were school aged. Dr. Cox's study in Great Britain looked at variations in both the material and cultural aspects of children's homes beginning when they were seven years of age in British Infant Schools. The children's educational attainments were followed until they were 15-years-old. Cox's findings support a complex theoretical model whereby the home environment's impact on later child achievement is mediated by parental support for school learning, as well as by child motivation, academic skill variables, and teacher attitudes.

Research by Drs. Bradley and Caldwell uses the HOME instrument which has been a powerful stimulant for research looking at home environments in terms of their potential for stimulating child cognitive advances. Their methodically painstaking attempts to parcel out the effects of parental processes (such as maternal acceptance, responsivity and involvement as well as provision of toys, organization and variety of home stimulation) reveal how powerful the effects of parental *contemporaneous* supports or lacks of support for academic achievement are when the school performance at age 11 is assessed in relation to earlier HOME measures when the child was six months, one, three, and four and one half years.

The critical importance of stability and continuity in parental supports for child learning is also emphasized by findings from research with male twins in Canada by Dr. Hugh Lytton and colleagues. By age nine, the best predictor for child cognitive ability was not maternal characteristics but level of earlier toddler vocabulary knowledge when the child was two. Maternal warmth and amount of time spent playing with her son also played a facilitative role in cognitive development of the nine-year-old boys. Such characteristics, of course, could *also* have fostered earlier speech development. Thus, although parental social practices at two years do not seem to predict directly very strongly, the indirect paths may be stronger.

Research by Drs. Leila Beckwith and Sarale Cohen focuses on an at-risk population of infants born prematurely whose development was followed for eight years. Neither the structural variable of social class *per se* nor the process variable of maternal responsivity in infancy alone predicted intellectual scores at eight years. By age eight, being reared in higher social class homes and in addition an above average responsive mothering experience in infancy were *both* necessary in order to produce high scoring, intellectually achieving youngsters.

Dr. Barnard and colleagues report on an innovative program to enhance very early parenting practices with infants. For almost a year, nurses visited mothers of premature infants with a specific curriculum to increase awareness of and responsiveness to infant states and signals. Early parenting practices were improved and parent-infant interactions heightened.

Focusing on another enrichment mode, Dr. Gotts reports on a longitudinal study of rural Appalachian families randomly assigned in preschool years to an educational television-only enrichment program for children versus an education television plus home visitation program that attempted to modify parental practices toward greater support for child academic achievement. After ten years, the home environment scores of parents who had received home visitor enrichment of their child development practices were significantly higher than scores of the parents of the television-only group. Although higher academic performance of the home-visitor group of children faded out after second grade, there was a strong indication that enhancing parenting skills to support academic achievement had worked. When school records were perused toward the end of secondary education, only 5% of the enriched parents' children had been held back in school at least one year while 25% of children without parental supports earlier had been held back in school at least one year. The HOME Environment Scale scores used to measure parental support for children's school learning reflected the positive effects of the home visitation program. Thus, correlations between social class and child achievement can be *attenuated* in low-education families as a function of parent education efforts to enhance family facilitation of child achievement.

The final paper in this collection by Dr. Earl Schaeffer supports a theoretical model that emphasizes the importance of "parental modernity" as evidenced by educational values and beliefs. Kindergarten teachers' ratings of child academic competence and child promotion to first grade were significantly correlated with measures of mother emotional and verbal responsiveness earlier during pregnancy and early infancy. "Modernity" reflects the positive effect of societal enlightenment and positive educational and occupational experiences, such that increased modernity of maternal scores is associated with higher child achievement. Child modernity achieved through educational means would also be expected, in turn, to have a positive impact on child competence.

The researches in this volume provide exciting food for thought. They increase our awareness of the necessity to measure not only structural variables such as family social class, but also process variables such as the interrelations, values, attitudes, and skills of parents as well as children in trying to predict child competence. These studies point to the importance of *continuity* of family support for cognitive competence, and also point to the subtle ways in which early responsive care can lead to early child cognitive/linguistic competence which can then predict later achievement. They challenge us to develop more subtle models to explain the pathways by which early parenting practices impact on later child achievement.

Reference

Honig, A.S. (1979). *Parent involvement in early childhood eduction*, Washington, DC: The National Association for the Education of Young Children.

Educational disadvantage: The bearing of the early home background on children's academic attainment and school progress

T. COX

University College of Swansea

This paper describes the result of a longitudinal study of a sample of children from culturally and materially disadvantaged homes and a matched control group in which the children's educational attainments were assessed at the ages of 7, 11 and 15 years respectively. The finding that the disadvantaged children made significantly poorer academic progress than their more advantaged peers throughout their entire school careers and appeared to suffer a 'cumulative deficit' in their academic learning, supports the view that the early home environment has a major bearing upon the child's subsequent school progress. However, the importance of the early environment in this respect is probably conditional upon the stability of that environment during the child's school years. Aspects of the early environment which may particularly bear upon the child's school progress are discussed, but the importance of the interplay between home, school and 'within child' factors in determining the child's academic attainment is acknowledged.

INTRODUCTION

Researchers have accumulated an overwhelming body of evidence in support of the view that the child's home background acts as a major determinant, or rather, set of determinants of his or her level of educational attainment and pattern of educational growth. Children from what might be termed culturally and materially disadvantaged homes tend, as a group, to under-achieve in schools compared wth more advantaged peers (Coleman, *et al.*, 1966; Plowden Report, 1957; Davie, *et al.*, 1972).

However, establishing the general importance of the home background for children's subsequent academic careers, in turn, raises a host of more specific questions concerning the manner and pattern of operation of the variables subsumed under this global heading. For example, at what stage in children's school careers do the effects of disadvantageous home background appear and in what aspects of educational progress and attainment are they most clearly manifest? Does the child's early home environment play a more crucial role in facilitating or retarding educational growth in school than the later home environment? What particular features of the home background are most closely associated with specific educational outcomes? Do disadvantaged children suffer a "cumulative deficit" in their learning as Deutsch (1965) proposed?

To answer these and related questions requires, ideally, longitudinal rather than cross-sectional research since the latter always suffers from the problem of the comparability of different age group samples, but longitudinal studies are relatively few in number due to their cost and practical and methodological difficulties. The largest and best known British longitudinal studies, which have covered the span of the compulsory school years are the National Survey of Health and Development (Douglas, *et al.*, 1968) and the National Child Development Study (Davie *et al.*, 1972, Fogelman *et al.*, 1978, Essen and Wedge, 1982.) There appear to be no comparable American studies of large representative samples of children conducted over a similar time span. No attempt will be made here to summarise the findings of these particular studies, or the light they throw upon some of the questions posed above, because of their sheer scope and complexity, although it can be said, in passing, that they offer general support for the major importance of the early home environment in shaping the course and outcome of children's educational development.

The intention of the present paper is to provide a synopsis of a longitudinal study carried out in Britain by the author which was designed to examine the effects of early cultural and material disadvantage in the home upon young children's subsequent school progress and adjustment and to explore some implications of its findings concerning the possible ways in which home background factors may influence children's academic development.

A LONGITUDINAL STUDY OF CULTURALLY DISADVANTAGED CHILDREN

The study was carried out in three stages:

Stage 1—The Original (Infant School) Study,

Stage 2—The First Follow-up Study (at age 11+ years),

Stage 3—The Second Follow-up Study (at age 15+ years).

For brevity, Stages 2 and 3 will be combined in the following account.

Stage 1: The Original (Infant School) Study

The study originated in the Schools Council's Research and Development Project in Compensatory Education based at Swansea University from 1967 to 1972. As part of that project an intensive study of a sub-sample of children attending infant schools in "deprived areas" in three cities in England and Wales was carried out. This sample comprised 52 children from homes judged to be disadvantaged on the basis of a structured parental interview in the home, the Disadvantaged Group (D.G.), and a comparison group of 52 children from more advantaged backgrounds, matched with the former group for age, sex, non-verbal reasoning (Raven's Coloured Progressive Matrices) and school, the Control Group (C.G.). Both groups were drawn from predominantly working class backgrounds. The parental interview was designed to yield four-point ratings of each home on five material and five cultural aspects of the home environment as follows:

Material Aspects
1. Income
2. Cleanliness of home
3. Quality of housing
4. Amount of play space (indoor and outdoor)
5. Mother's health and stability

Cultural Aspects
6. Mother's education
7. Social class grouping of father's occupation
8. Availability and suitability of play materials and books
9. Provision of cultural experiences (television viewing, outings, etc.)
10. Level of parental interest in the child's educational development

The ratings of the material and cultural factors were added to provide total Material and Cultural scores which, in turn, were combined to yield a total Home Background score upon which the final selection of the children for the sample was based. The sample was drawn up toward the end of the children's first school year when they were aged approximately 5½ years, and studied over the two remaining infant school years. The study concentrated on linguistic and related educational skills but within a comprehensive scheme of assessment. Data from individual or group tests were supplemented by teachers' ratings of the children's concepts and skills in language, reading and mathematics and also of their school behaviour and attitudes, including motivation and concentration.

It was found that, from the outset of the study, the D.G. children consistently performed less well than their C.G. peers on a wide range of linguistic and scholastic measures and were judged by their teachers to be less well adjusted socially and emotionally to school and to show poorer concentration in school activities. Toward the end of their infant school careers (i.e. ages 7½ to 8 years) the disadvantaged children were significantly more retarded in reading and spelling than their C.G. peers in relation to their age group. It was concluded that poor educational home conditions adversely affected children's development in school, particularly in the "basic" scholastic skills of reading, spelling and number and in certain oral language skills. (For a full report on this study see Chazan et al., 1977.)

Stages 2 and 3: The Follow-up Studies

The present author carried out two follow-up studies of the Disadvantaged and Control Group children. The first of these, funded by the Schools Council, took place when the children were aged approximately 11½ years and spanned their final primary school term and their first secondary school term. The second follow-up study, funded by the Social Science Research Council, was begun when the children were aged approximately 15½ years and spanned the final term of their fourth secondary school year and the whole of their fifth school year. These two follow-up studies, sequence may become increasingly backward as time goes on when compared with children making normal progress, since their initial handicap may impair later learning, producing a cumulative deficit in the learning curve unless effective and timely remedial measures are taken. Evidence to support this view came from the results of a multiple regression analysis carried out on the *combined* C.G. and D.G. samples ($N = 92$) aimed at finding the best combination of early (6–7 years) predictors of later (15 + year) reading attainment.

Eight predictor variables (see Table II) were selected from the original (infant school) study data on the basis of their likely casual bearing upon future scholastic progress and their relatively low inter-correlations. The criterion variable was a measure of reading attainment at age 15½ years approximately (N.F.E.R Reading Attainment Test EHl). The results are presented in Table III which shows that nearly two-thirds (64%) of the variance in 15 + year reading test scores was accounted for by a combination of five predictor variables, with reading test score at age 7 years emerging as the best single predictor, accounting for 41% of the variance. However, the addition of four other predictors namely, home background (total rating), receptive vocabulary, non-verbal reasoning and task orientation improved the prediction by a further 23%. In fact, when a further regression analysis was carried out *omitting* seven year reading score these four variables between them accounted for 57% of the 15 year reading test variance, i.e. nearly as much as when the early reading score was included. Clearly then, these particular variables are important in their own right as well as in combination with early reading test score. Indeed, they may well have played a major role in determining initial reading performance. (Except for vocabulary, these variables also contributed significantly to the prediction of 5+ year attainment in spelling and mathematics, in combination with 7 year attainment test score in those subjects.)

It seems likely that the children's early home environment had a major influence upon the children's later academic attainment (reading), both indirectly through its influence upon *early* attainment, which, in turn, was linked to later attainment levels and, directly, perhaps, through influencing children's attitudes and

TABLE II
Infant School Variables Selected to Predict
Children's Reading Attainment at 15+ Years

Variable	Content
1. Burt Graded Word Reading Test Score (7½ years)	World reading (oral)
2. English Picture Vocabulary Test 1 score (7 years)	Oral receptive vocabulary
3. Story retelling task score (6½ years)	Oral fluency/expressiveness
4. Raven's Coloured Progressive Matrices (7 years)	Non-verbal (perceptual) reasoning
5. Social Hostility (irritability and resentfulness) score (7 years)	Two of three component factors of the Schaefer Classroom Behaviour Inventory*
6. Task Orientation (perseverance and concentration) score (7 years)	
7. Percentage average school attendance over the three infant school years	—
8. Total score on parental home interview schedule (material and cultural factors) (6 years)	Home background

NOTE: Ages in brackets show the children's mean age for each variable.

* This unpublished inventory comprised 60 child behaviour items, each to be rated on a four-point scale by the class teacher. The overall scores are expressed in terms of three major dimensions, Social Hostility, Task Orientation and Extraversion.

motivation towards reading and their confidence in themselves as learners; attitudes that may well have been sustained during subsequent years. Moreover, the original designation of the groups of children as "Disadvantaged" or "Control" was based, in part, upon the extent to which their homes engendered an interest in and knowledge of literacy through the provision of suitable books for

TABLE III

Prediction of 15 + Year Reading Test Score From Selected 6 to 7 Year Measures (Control and Disadvantaged Groups Combined) in a Multiple Regression Analysis ($N = 80$)

Step	Predictor Variable	F to Enter	Signif.	Multiple R	R^2	R^2 Change	Simple R	Overall F
1	Reading	52.00	0.00	0.64	0.41	0.41	0.64	52.00
2	Home background	19.61	0.00	0.73	0.54	0.12	0.57	42.42
3	Oral vocabulary	10.29	0.00	0.77	0.60	0.06	0.58	35.36
4	Non-verbal reasoning	5.85	0.02	0.79	0.63	0.03	0.46	29.79
5	Task orientation	2.74	0.10	0.80	0.64	0.01	0.49	24.97
6	School attendance	0.64	0.43	0.80	0.65	0.00	0.19	20.81
7	Oral fluency	0.87	0.35	0.81	0.65	0.00	0.47	17.93
8	Social hostility	0.21	0.65	0.81	0.65	0.00	0.29	15.53

NOTES: 1. Seven year reading scores were unavailable for 12 of the 92 children in the total sample.
2. The dependent variable in the above multiple regression analysis was a measure of reading attainment at 15 + years (N.F.E.R. Reading Test EHI).

the children and adults in the home reading to the children or hearing them read. Other recent British studies (Wells, in press, Hewison and Tizard, 1980) have clearly identified the central importance of this literacy factor in the home in determining children's subsequent reading performance in school.

However, it is not clear from the evidence provided by the present study to what extent the significance of the home background as a long term predictor of reading achievement, over and above its contribution to early reading achievement, derives from the fact that the early home background measures proved to be stable over most of the children's school careers, so that the early home influences upon children's patterns of learning were sustained over subsequent years. This is a theoretical issue which has been addressed by other researchers. Gottfried (1984), summarising a group of longitudinal studies in the U.S.A. which examined the relationship between aspects of the home environment and very young children's cognitive development, stated that most of the findings he reviewed supported the view that early home environment related to later intellectual development because of the stability of that environment. Such a conclusion accords well with the position of Clarke and Clarke (1976) who argue that, when considering the role of early cultural deprivation in children's cognitive development, it is vital to consider the nature of the child's learning experiences *following* the deprivation since this may prolong what might otherwise be only transitory adverse effects on such development. On this view cumulative deficit in learning will occur only where the child remains in a learning environment lacking sufficient intellectual stimulus and guidance. However, this view seems to take no account of the possibly cumulative effects of early failure in a learning sequence discussed earlier in this paper.

Regarding the specific aspects of the home environment showing the highest correlations with measures of young children's cognitive performance, Gottfried reported that these were measures of maternal involvement with the child, provision of appropriate play materials and opportunities for variety in daily stimulation and it is interesting to note that these or similar aspects were included in the together with the original (infant school) study, thus constituted a logitudinal study of the children's progress and achievement throughout their entire school careers up to the end of the period of compulsory school education in Britain.

By the second follow-up study the sample size had dropped to 46 D.G. and 46 C.G. children. In both follow-up studies the children's homes were revisited and re-appraised on the home background rating scales used in the original study, modified to take account of the children's increased age. At both ages, 11+ and 15+ years, the D.G. children remained significantly disadvantaged in relation to their C.G. peers in terms of their home backgrounds, apart to one or two individual cases where family circumstances had changed. The cultural and material disadvantage they experienced thus lasted throughout their childhood and early adolescence. The Disadvantaged and Control Groups remained matched for age and sex, and reasonably well matched for non-verbal reasoning ability (although the C.G. children showed a slight superiority) but, as was to be expected, the originally close matching for school had broken down somewhat by the age of 11 years and subsequently. Even so there was still a substantial overlap between the two groups in terms of primary and secondary schools they attended and it could be claimed that the loss of control of "the school" variable was not so great that it seriously undermined the research design in its focus upon the influece of home background factors.

The assessment programme was broadly similar for both follow-up studies and included the completion of self report scales by the pupils on their self concepts and academic motivation as well as a wide range of linguistic and educational attainment tests and teacher ratings of the children's attainments and social and emotional adjustment to school. The pattern of findings from the two studies was broadly similar with the most pronounced differences between the Control and Disadvantaged Groups appearing in the area of basic educational attainment (reading, essay writing, spelling and mathematics), and lesser (though in many cases still statistically significant) differences in the areas of oral language skills and personality (self esteem and academic motivation). In contrast to their C.G. peers, only a handful of D.G.

children attained a minimal level of formal educational qualifications at age 16+ years (i.e. in G.C.E. 'O' level or C.S.E. examinations), and the majority of them left school at that age and did not enter full time further education or training, so that their career prospects were markedly poorer than those of their more advantaged peers.

Since some of the educational attainment tests had been administered to the sample at three stages in their school careers, 7+, 11+ and 15+ years, it was possible to analyse the data for evidence of a "cumulative deficit" in the performance of the D.G. children relative to their C.G. peers. Such evidence was found insofar as the differences in attainment between the two groups at 11 and 15 years respectively were greater than would have been predicted on the basis of their earlier scores on the same or similar tests, although some of the differences failed to reach statistical significance (Cox, 1983).

Despite some loss of control of factors in the matched group design over time, the findings from the two follow-up studies support the conclusion that disadvantageous home conditions can have a long term depressing influence upon children's academic progress and attainment and a correspondingly adverse affect upon their social and emotional adjustment and attitude to school, and subsequent career prospects (Cox, 1982, Cox and Jones, 1983). In general, the Disadvantaged Group children did not come from the most severely disadvantaged homes because they were selectively screened for non-verbal reasoning ability in the original study and the urban areas from which their infant schools were selected were not the decaying inner areas of large cities where deprivation and family stresses are probably most acute. However, in the general population moderately disadvantaged families will outnumber the more severely impoverished ones and the present study showed that even moderately disadvantageous home conditions can significantly impair children's school progress.

THE INFLUENCE OF THE EARLY HOME ENVIRONMENT

Given that the home conditions of the children in this study, whether advantaged as disadvantaged, remained fairly stable between the ages of approximately 6 and 15 years it seems likely that the relevant home background factors were acting in a *sustained* fashion to influence the children's educational performance. Does this mean that early home conditions can only have a long term influence upon children's academic attainment if they are sustained over the child's formative years, as in the present study? Further, what specific aspects of the early home background appear to be most influential upon children's academic attainment? The study was not specially designed to examine these questions but the data it yielded may offer at least some partial answers to them.

Regarding the long term influence of the early home background it was clear that the latter had an immediate impact upon the children's school performance, causing the Disadvantaged Group children to fall behind their C.G. peers in vital aspects of educational functoning, and, as will be demonstrated shortly, the children's early level of attainment was positively related to later achievement levels. Nowhere is this seen more clearly than in the case of progress in reading which is fundamental to the whole formal educational process. At intervals during the three full years of the sample children's infant school careers, their teachers recorded each child's level on the basic reading scheme used in the school, a crude but reasonably valid index of reading progress. Table I shows clearly that, as early as the end of the first year, the D.G. children were lagging significantly behind their C.G. peers on this measure and remained in this adverse position during the following two years.

This result was supported by the finding of a significant difference between the two groups, in favour of the Control Group, on a standardised reading test (Burt Graded Word Reading Test) given to the children during their second and third infant school years. A similar pattern emerged in the case of the children's progress in mathematical skills and concepts, as rated by their infant school teachers, and also in writing and spelling skills. The development of skill in the "3Rs" follows a more or less hierarchical progression in which higher-order skills are built upon more fundamental lower order skills. Thus, children who start the learning cycle with a relatively poor grasp of the earliest skills in the

TABLE I

Children's Reading Scheme Level at the Infant School Stage

Reading Scheme Level	End of first year				End of second year				End of third year			
	C.G. (N=52)		D.G. (N=52)		C.G. (N=52)		D.G. (N=52)		C.G. (N=46)		D.G. (N=46)	
	N	%	N	%	N	%	N	%	N	%	N	%
1. Pre-reading	8	15	16	31	0	0	4	8	0	0	1	2
2. Introductory Book/Book 1	25	48	22	42	9	17	16	31	1	2	7	15
3. Book 2/3	13	25	12	23	21	40	18	35	12	26	18	39
4. Book 4 or beyond	6	11	2	4	17	33	14	27	18	39	14	30
5. Beyond basic reading scheme	0	0	0	0	5	10	0	0	15	33	6	13

NOTE: On each occasion there was a statistically significant different between the Control and Disadvantaged Groups in the proportions of children falling into the five categories (Kendall's Tau).

KEY: C.G.: Control Group
     D.G.: Disadvantaged Group

ratings of the children's home backgrounds used in the present study.

It has already been argued that the early home background may have had a major influence upon another of the effective early predictors of later reading performances, namely the measure of reading at 7 years. It may well be that, in a similar fashion, two of the remaining three useful predictors, receptive vocabulary and task orientation also reflect the direct influence of the home background. The scope of the child's receptive oral vocabulary at age 7 would obviously be at least partly determined by the quality of the experiences provided in the early home background and, especially, by the quality of the verbal interaction between the parent(s) and the child in relation to those experiences. In like manner, the child's motivation toward and ability to concentrate on the structured learning tasks typically provided in school (positive task orientation) would be shaped by the extent of his experience of similar learning tasks in the home and the degree of parental encouragement to pursue them. The third useful predictor, non-verbal reasoning, may also be partly influenced by the quality of the child's early home experiences but, since the particular measure of this ability used is often claimed to be relatively culture free (Raven, 1981), the extent of such influence is probably less than is the case with the afore mentioned predictor variables.

OTHER MAJOR DETERMINANTS OF ACADEMIC ACHIEVEMENT

Although early home background factors clearly play a major role in determining children's initial educational attainment and their effects may extend to achievement in the later school years in the ways already discussed it would be foolish to claim that they are the only important factors impinging upon children's educational progress and achievement. As Clarke (1984) points out there has been a good deal of recent methodologically sophisticated research indicating the importance of school and teacher variables as factors

bearing upon children's academic and general educational progress (See Rutter, 1983, for a summary). By the very nature of its
design the longitudinal study of disadvantaged pupils carried out
by the present writer tried to exclude the operation of such factors
in order to highlight the influence of home background factors but
some loss of control in this respect at later stages in the study has
already been acknowledged.

Despite the highly significant mean differences in the academic
attainments, at different ages, of the Disadvantaged and Control
Groups in this study there was, in fact, a good deal of overlap
between the two groups at the individual level. This finding clearly
supports the view that the child's home background is not the only
determinant of children's school progress and adjustment. That is,
coming from a "good" home does not guarantee academic success
any more than coming from a "poor" home inevitably leads to low
academic attainment, despite the positive general correlation
between home background and achievement. In a report on the
first follow-up study (Cox & Jones, 1983) the writers discussed the
important but relatively little researched questions of why some
children from disadvantaged homes flourish educationally whilst
some from more advantageous homes do rather poorly. Case
studies illustrating such exceptions to the generally positive link
between background and achievement were explored and their
possible implications discussed.

One of these cases, Peter, illustrates how a child from a
classically disadvantaged background may sometimes achieve
scholastic success against all apparent odds. He came from a large
family living in grossly overcrowded conditions in a poorly
decorated and furnished flat with a long term unemployed father
and a stressed, apathetic mother. There were few children's books
in evidence and only a meagre supply of toys but the father
appeared to take an interest in the children and read to Peter at
least occasionally. The general level of cultural provision in this
poverty stricken family was very low although the children did
watch television regularly.

Peter had not attended nursery school but settled quickly into his
infant school where, on entry, he could write his name legibly and

draw simple recognisable objects. During his three years at the school he appeared to be well adjusted, concentrating well on tasks that interested him and making steady scholastic progress. At age 7+ years he had advanced beyond the basic reading scheme, showing a fairly keen interest in reading and a good grasp of number concepts and operations, and he scored at around the nine year level on standardised reading and spelling tests. He continued this good academic progress through his junior school although he was described at age eleven years as a rather withdrawn child who was difficult to get to know. According to tests administered at 7 and 11 years his non-verbal reasoning ability was above average.

It would seem that, despite his family's poverty and bad living conditions and lack of suitable books and play materials, an interest in reading and other educational activities had somehow been kindled in this child and this may have been sustained by his above-average level of (non-verbal) cognitive ability. As he was a somewhat withdrawn, "hard to reach" child, it seems unlikely that his good academic progress depended upon a supportive personal relationship with his teachers although, of course, he may have responded to the more general learning atmosphere of the classroom. In Peter's case it seems that his motivation to learn in school was primarily self-determined but this, in turn, would evoke a positive response and interest from his teachers and, possibly, his parents, which would further assist the learning process.

This case, together with others described by the writers, illustrate that the determinants of a pupil's educational growth do not lie exclusively within the child's external environment, whether his home, school or local or wider culture, but also exist within the child himself in the form of his unique pattern of cognitive abilities, personality and motivation which, itself, is the result of the interaction between innate and environmental factors. In other words, children are not merely the passive recipients of environmental forces but may actually help to shape them. Such an interactionist viewpoint has come to be known as the transactional model of development, according to which there are continuous interactions across the years of development between the developing organism and the social/educational environment, in which mutual feedback plays an important part (Clarke, 1984, Schweinhart & Weikart, 1980), although Gottfried (1984) subsumes such organism-environment interaction into a general systems theory model. This stresses the importance of individual differences in children, for example, with respect to their responsivity to stimulation and the types of stimulation they seek out. A further principle of the theory, termed evocative 'genotype-environment interaction', proposes that different child characteristics elicit different responses from the social and physical environment.

All of these home environment variables coexist with a range of other major factors bearing upon the child's educational progress in school, including school and teacher variables and "within child" factors which interact with the child's home and school environment and, indeed, help to shape it. The way in which these various environmental and intrinsic factors may interact to shape the course of the child's academic development is illustrated in Figure 1. This is an empirical/clinical rather than a theoretically based model although it accepts the organism-environment interaction postulate of the transactional and general systems theory of child development. It focuses exclusively upon the contribution of home and school environmental factors but the fact that the concept of the child's environment could be extended to include neighbourhood and wider socio-cultural influences is acknowledged (Gottfried, 1984).

SUMMARY AND CONCLUSION

The longitudinal study described above supports the view that the quality of educational experience and provision in the child's early home background is a major determinant of the child's level of early academic attainment in school, and, to some extent, of subsequent academic achievement, provided that the home environment remains stable over time. Probably the most fundamentally important feature of the early home environment is the general degree of interest and involvement shown by the parents or caregivers in the child's educational and general growth. This will

FIGURE 1   Some Determinants of Children's Early Academic Achievement: an Empirical Model

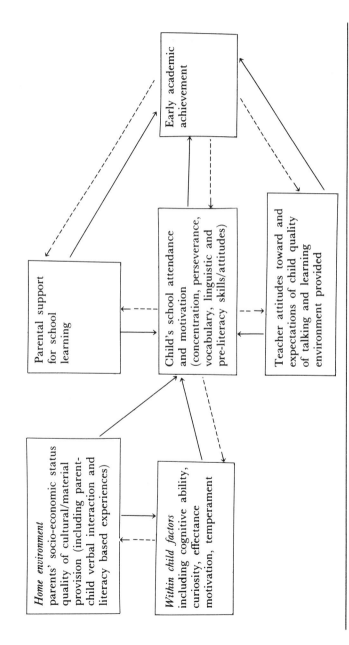

PRE-SCHOOL STAGE

EARLY SCHOOL CAREER

Home environment
parents' socio-economic status
quality of cultural/material
provision (including parent-
child verbal interaction and
literacy based experiences)

Within child factors
including cognitive ability,
curiosity, effectance
motivation, temperament

Parental support
for school
learning

Child's school attendance
and motivation
(concentration, perseverance,
vocabulary, linguistic and
pre-literacy skills/attitudes)

Early academic
achievement

Teacher attitudes toward and
expectations of child quality
of talking and learning
environment provided

NOTE: Continuous lines indicate suggested direction of causality and hatched lines interaction be manifest growth, including the degree of literacy knowledge and interest cultivated in the home, the quality of verbal interaction between parent and child and the fostering of children's intellectual curiosity through structured learning experiences.

This paper has not directly addressed the implications of the research findings described for educational or socio-economic intervention designed to combat the deleterious effects of cultural material disadvantage in the home upon children's academic achievement and progress. However, in that these findings underline the importance of the child's early learning experiences at home and at school in establishing patterns of later academic development they lend strong support to the principles of mounting such intervention *as early as possible* and sustaining it, at least at intervals, during the subsequent years of childhood, and of helping parents to achieve an active, supportive role, with teachers, in the process of educating the child. It is the function of "action orientated" research to explore the most effective ways of delivering appropriate educational and socio-economic intervention.

Acknowledgements

The writer wishes to acknowledge the generous support of the Schools Council which funded the first follow-up study and the Social Science Research Council which funded the second follow-up study.

References

Chazan, M., Cox, T., Jackson, S. & Laing, A.F. (1977). *Studies of Infant School Children, Volume 2, Deprivation and Development,* Oxford: Basil Blackwell for the Schools Council.

Clarke, A.M., & Clarke, A.D.B. (1976). *Early Experience: Myth and Evidence,* London: Open Books.

Clarke, A.M. (1984). Early Experience and Cognitive Development, *Review of Research in Education,* 11, 125–57.

Coleman, J.S., Campbell, E.Q., Hobson, C.J., McPartland, J., Mood, A.M., Weinfeld, F.D., & York, R.L. (1966). *Equality of Educational Opportunity,* Washington, D.C.: U.S. Government Printing Office.

Cox, T. (1982). Disadvantaged Fifteen-year-olds: initial findings from a longitudinal study, *Educ. Studies,* 8, 1–13.

Cox, T. (1983). Cumulative deficit in culturally disadvantaged children, *Brit. J. Educ. Psychol.,* 53, 317–26.

Cox, T., & Jones, G. (1983). *Disadvantaged 11-Year-Olds. Book Supplement to the Journal of Child Psychology and Psychiatry, No. 3*, Oxford: Pergamon Press.

Davie, R., Butler, N. & Goldstein, H. (1972). *From Birth to Seven. The Second Report of the National Child Development Study (1968 Cohort)*, London: Longman in association with the National Children's Bureau.

Deutsch, M. (1965). The role of social class in language development and cognition, *Amer. J. Orthopsychiat.*, **35,** 78–88.

Douglas, J.W.B., Ross, J.M. & Simpson, H.R. (1968) *All Our Future*, London: Davies.

Essen, J. & Wedge, P. (1982). *Continuities in Childhood Disadvantage*, London: Heineman.

Fogelman, K.R., Goldstein, H., Essen, J & Ghodsian, M. (1978). Patterns of attainment, *Educ. Studies*, **4,** 121–30.

Gottfried, A.W. (Ed.) (1984). *Home Environment and Early Cognitive Development: Logitudinal Research*, New York: Academic Press.

Hewison, J. & Tizard, J. (1980). Parental involvement and reading attainment, *Brit. J. Educ. Psychol.*, **50,** 209–15.

Plowden Report. (1967). Central Advisory Council for Education (England). *Children and their Primary Schools Volume 1: Report, Volume 2: Research and Surveys*, London: H.M.S.O.

Raven, J. (1981). *Manual for Raven's Progressive Matrices and Mill Hill Vocabulary Scales*, Research Supplement No. 1, London: H.K. Lewis.

Rutter, M. (1983). School effects on pupil progress: research findings and policy implications, *Child Development*, **54,** 1–29.

Schweinhart, L.J., & Weikart, D.P. (1980). *Young Children Grow up: The Effects of the Perry Pre-school Program on Youths through Age 15*. Monograph of the High/Scope Educational Research Foundation. Ypsilanti, M.I.: High Scope Press.

Wells, C.G. (in press). Pre-school literacy activities and success in school. In Olsen, D. *et al.* (eds.), *The Nature and Consequences of Literacy*, Cambridge: Cambridge University Press.

Social Interaction with the parent during infancy and later intellectual competence in children born preterm

LEILA BECKWITH and SARALE E. COHEN

University of California at Los Angeles

Maternal caregiving and social interaction patterns were assessed for 55 prematurely born infants at 1, 8, and 24 months. Mothers were considered more responsive if they scored above the median on 2 of the 3 home visit observations. Gesell Developmental Schedules were given to the children at 24 months, Stanford-Binet at age 5 and WISC-R at age 8 years. At each age period through 8 years, children whose caregivers had been socially responsive in infancy had cognitive scores superior to those of children whose caregivers were less socially responsive in infancy. By age 8 years, being reared in a higher social class home was insufficient by itself, as was a good infant-mother relationship, to produce high cognitive scores. Both factors were necessary to result in intellectually competent children.

Research indicates that the early home invironment is significantly associated with later intellectual competence. The relationship has been found in diverse groups, that is, in low as well as middle-income families, in several ethnic groups, and in biologically at risk as well as non-risk children (Bradley & Caldwell, 1976; Clarke-Stewart, 1973; Gottfried, 1984; Moore, 1968). Within these groups, aspects of the animate and inanimate environment provided by the family appear either to enhance or interfere with later cognitive functioning. The present report will illustrate our work derived from a longitudinal study of preterm infants and their families who have been studied from birth to eight years of age (Cohen, Parmelee, Sigman, & Beckwith, in press). In this paper, we shall examine the relations between one aspect of the child's early experience in the home, that is social interactions between parent and child during infancy, and intelligence test scores at school age, at ages five and eight.

Preterm children differing in gestational age, birthweight, perinatal risk and social class background were selected in order to

B

determine whether early social experience can act as an ameliora-
tive factor to reduce adverse developmental consequences often
associated with perinatal complications. The rapid increase of
medical technology and medical knowledge allows more infants to
survive and with fewer major sensory and motor handicaps, yet,
there is evidence that such children show an increased incidence of
learning problems at school age (Davies, 1984).

During early infancy, preterm infants, as a group, differ from
term healthy infants in motor patterns, state organization, and
visual attention (Kopp, 1984). Their parents are more likely than
are parents of term healthy infants to experience increased grief,
anxiety, and guilt about their infants' birth and development
(Minde, 1980). During social interaction preterm infants and their
parents show less joy and less pleasure in interaction with each
other than do term infants with their parents (Goldberg, 1983).

We have focused on one aspect of parent-child social interaction,
that is responsive and reciprocal social interaction, as it affects later
global cognitive functioning. The degree to which the infant
experienced responsive and reciprocal social interaction was
assessed directly by time sampling that noted the frequency of
specific social interactions during multiple cross-time home
observations. Although rating scales of parental sensitivity and
responsiveness have proven to be very effective measuring tools
(Ainsworth, Blehar, Waters, & Wall, 1978) we chose a method that
enabled us to describe more concretely what actually occurred.

Many studies have shown that global descriptors of the parents'
own characteristics, their education and social class, relate to
children's intelligence test performance. Most studies find that
children with more educated mothers and/or children with middle
class parents show higher IQ scores than children with less
educated and/or lower class parents (Deutsch, 1973). Those
relations are probably mediated by both genetic and environmental
forces. It has been contended that genetic factors contribute
significantly to the relation between the home environment and
children's intelligence (Scarr, 1981). It has also been established
that more educated and/or higher social status parents provide

their children with a home environment that is more intellectually stimulating (Deutsch, 1973).

The question therefore can be asked, if an association is found between early social experience and later cognitive development, is it a direct relation or is the association spuriously due to factors of maternal education or family social class, factors related to both the nature of the social interactions and the nature of the cognitive development. In order to pinpoint the importance of proximal events of early social experience, it is important to distinguish those events from confounding distal factors. We have attempted to do so in this paper.

METHOD

Sample

The children described in this report were all born preterm at the hospital at the University of California in Los Angeles or were transferred soon after birth to the Neonatal Intensive care Unit at the hospital. All preterm infants in the nursery were potential subjects for the study and were enrolled in the study if they were born at a gestational age of 37 weeks or less and with a birthweight equal to or less than 2500 grams and were free of major sensory or motor handicaps in the perinatal period. All infants included in the study were born between July 1972 and December 1974.

A total of 126 preterm infants were followed until age 2 years; 100 through 5 years and 93 until 8 years. The group was composed of English speaking families and several immigrant groups whose primary language was not English. We have previously reported differences, beginning at age 2 and continuing through age 8, in cognitive scores from children whose families were not fluent in English. Because of those differences, analyses are done according to the language group of the family (Cohen & Parmelee, 1983).

For the current paper we selected a subsample of 55 children that fulfilled the following requirements:

1. came from families where English was the primary language spoken in the home;
2. lived with their biological mother, at least for the first two years of life when the three home assessments were made.
3. and had shown no major handicaps of a sensory or motor nature in their testing at 2, 5, or 8 years.

As infants they varied in the number of biological hazards they suffered. A number of the infants were very sick and had long hospitalizations whereas some of the children had a relatively benign health course. As a group, they were somewhat heavier, older, and less sick than a comparable sample today. As neonates, 56% were considered to have respiratory distress of whom 18% received ventilatory assistance. No infant had bronchopulmonary dysplasia. There was no information at that time as to intraventricular hemmorhages.

The group was heterogeneous as to social backgrounds with parental occupations varying from unskilled laborers to physicians. The Hollingshead 4 factor index (1975) was used to describe the family's social economic status. It is based on the educational and occupational status of both parents. On the average, the sample was lower—middle class. Table I presents a summary description of the biological and demographic characteristics of the sample. At 8 year follow-up testing 65% of the children were living with their original nuclear family and 63% of the mothers were employed.

Measures

Home Environment, Measures of Responsive Caregiving: Assessments of the infant's caregiving experience were made during three naturalistic home observations in which specific social transactions were noted. The observations were made at 1, 8, and 24 months after the infant's expected date of birth by one of a pool of four observers. At each observation, frequencies of specific discrete behaviors were noted every 15 seconds on precoded checklists or by event sampling. The one month visit in the home consisted of an observation through a cycle of the baby's waking up from sleep, a

TABLE I
Summary of Sample Description (N = 55)

	Mean	Range
Gestational age—weeks	32.3	25–37
Birthweight—grams	1802.8	800–2495
Length of hospitalization—days	28.5	2–88
Maternal age—years	25.7	16–39
Maternal education—years	13.0	8–17
Hollingshead index—4 factors	44.4	19–66
Obstetrical complications[a]	82.1	50–112
Postnatal complications[a]	87.8	55–160
% Boys	58	
% Firstborn	55	

[a]Scale was standardized on full-term infants so as to have a M of 100 and SD of 20. A high score is optimal.

feeding time, and all caregiving and other activities that occurred until the baby was asleep for more than 1/2 hour. The average awake time at the 1 month observation was 74 minutes. At the 8 month visit, the observation consisted of 90 minutes of awake time plus a feeding. At the 24 month visit continuous event sampling was done for 50 minutes of play time. A more complete description of the procedure and the categories, and the observer reliability can be found in previous publications (Beckwith and Cohen, 1984).

At each age a large number of individual behaviors were observed. In order to characterize the caregiving at each age period we have devised a summary score based on a priori selected social behaviors which are responsive to the baby's signals of gaze, vocalization, smile or gesture. For the current paper we have focused on the social environment and have not included any measures of the inanimate environment or asocial aspects of the caregiving environment that have been reported in previous publications. The behaviors selected at one month were (1) the percent of the baby's awake time in which the mother provided social interaction with the baby by holding, touching, talking or mutual gazing; (2) the percent of awake time in which the mother and baby were in the *en face* position; (3) the percent of time during which the mother talked to the baby in the *en face* position; (4) the percentage of fussing or crying episodes of the baby to which the mother responded positively within 45 seconds. At 8 months the variables that were selected were similar, except that the mother's vocal imitation or response to the baby's nondistress vocalization was included, rather than the mother's contingent response to the baby's distress. Two variables were selected at 24 months as analogues to the variables at 1 and 8 months; 1) the amount of social interaction the mother engaged in with the child by touching, talking, or presenting a toy, and 2) the degree of which either the child or the mother responded to each other verbally as in a conversational exchange, or nonverbally as in reciprocal play such as rolling a ball back and forth.

Social behaviors at each age period were converted to standardized scores and then summed. The sums were then standardized to make a single composite score per observation for each caregiver-child dyad. Table II presents the components of the summary score of responsive caregiving for each of the three age periods.

TABLE II
Components of Responsive Caregiving Summary Score

1 Month	8 Months	24 Months
Attentiveness	Attentiveness	Attentiveness
Mutual visual regard	Mutual visual regard	
Face-to-face talk	Face-to-face talk	Reciprocal interactions
Contingency to distress	Contingency to vocalization	

COGNITIVE DEVELOPMENT

Each child's developmental status was assessed longitudinally by independent testers who were unaware of the home observation data. At 24 months, a pediatrician administered the Gesell Developmental Schedules. The Stanford-Binet, From L was given by a psychologist at 5 years and the Wechsler-Intelligence Scale for Children, Revised Form was given by a different psychologist at 8 years.

RESULTS

We have followed the sample from birth through 8 years of age. In the current analyses we will examine the relation of the social environment in infancy, as measured by responsive caregiving, to later cognitive development. We will then examine those variables that are associated with responsive caregiving and attempt to determine what appears to mediate the relationship between responsive caregiving and cognitive development.

Question 1. Was responsive caregiving associated with cognitive development?

In order to test the relationship between responsive caregiving and cognitive development, and to take advantage of the multiple assessments made, we divided the sample at the median into more and less responsive caregiving on the basis of the caregiving scores obtained during the three home visits. For each home visit the scores were divided at the median into more or less responsive. A mother then could have anywhere between zero and three responsive caregiving scores. Those caregivers who had a responsive caregiving summary score above the median on 2 or 3 of the home observations, regardless of the sequence of caregiving over time, were considered more responsive (N = 28) and those whose responsive caregiving score was below the median on 2 or 3 of the home visits were considered as less responsive (N = 27). Eleven mothers (20%) never achieved a single responsive caregiving score.

Sixteen mothers (29%) were responsive one of the three visits, a score that could be attained by being more responsive than the median at any one of the visits. The most common pattern of only one responsive score, however, was to be responsive at one month, but not to be able to maintain the responsiveness, the "turn off" phenomenon. Thirteen mothers (24%) were responsive two of the three visits. Within this group the most common pattern was to become responsive after the one month visit, that is to "turn onto" the infant. An approximately equal number of mothers "turned on" as "turned off". Fifteen mothers (27%) were consistently responsive all three visits.

The cognitive development of the children was then examined at 2, 5, and 8 years by univariate t tests. The results for each age interval are summarized in Table III. The univariate t test values are as follows: 2 years $t = 2.56$, p<.05; 5 years $t = 2.17$, p<.01; and 8 years $t = 2.26$, p<.05. At each age period through age 8 years the children of caregivers socially responsive in infancy did significantly better than did children whose caregivers were less socially responsive in infancy.

TABLE III
Cognitive Development and Responsive Caregiving

	Less Responsive	More Responsive
Gesell—24 months		
M	98.2*	105.6
S.D.	9.2	12.1
Stanford-Binet—5 Years		
M	98.8**	110.8
S.D.	18.6	11.4
WISC-R-8 Years		
M	104.3*	113.6
S.D.	15.4	15.1

*p<.05
**p<.01

Question 2. What promoted or affected responsive caregiving? The next sets of analyses were directed at examining differences between caregivers who were responsive and those who were less responsive. A series of *t* tests were done on variables describing neonatal medical status and demographic variables. These analyses are summarized in Table IV. The two responsivity groups did not differ on any of the variables that related to the neonatal medical status of the infant nor on the mother's obstetrical course. In contrast, the responsivity groups differed on demographic variables. The more responsive mothers were likely to have firstborn

TABLE IV

Comparison of Caregiving Groups on Neonatal Status and Demographic Variables

| | Caregiving | | | |
| | Less Responsive N = 27 | | More Responsive N = 28 | |
	Mean	S.D.	Mean	S.D.
Gestational age—weeks	32.4	3.3	32.0	3.5
Birthweight—grams	1833.4	522.3	1773.3	527.2
Length of hospitalization —days	27.0	24.7	30.0	22.0
Maternal age —years	25.5	6.1	25.8	4.4
Maternal education —years	12.3	1.7*	13.8	2.2
Hollingshead index	39.5	11.3*	49.1	13.8
Obstetrical complications[a]	82.6	15.9	81.6	14.1
Postnatal complications[a]	88.6	32.2	87.1	28.6
% Boys	53		47	
% Firstborn	29	*	71	

*$p<.01$
[a]High score is optimal

children. $\chi^2 = 9.6$, p<.01). Those mothers who were responsive were more educated than were mothers who were less responsive ($t = 2.71$, p<.01) and had a higher social class Hollingshead Index ($t = 2.80$, p<.01). Thus, social, not biological factors, appeared to promote responsive caregiving.

Question 3:   Did birth order, maternal education, or social class by themselves explain the relationship between responsive caregiving and cognitive development?

Sets of 2 × 2 analyses of variance were conducted to test the differences in cognitive development as a function of more or less responsive caregiving coupled with variables that were shown to be associated with it, namely, birth order, maternal education, and social class.

Table V presents the scores on developmental tests at 2, 5, and 8 years according to birth order and responsive caregiving. Although whether a child is first or later born is related to the quality of social responsiveness of the mother, neither birth order nor responsive

TABLE V

Cognitive Development Secores Related to Responsive Caregiving and Birth Order

	Less Responsive		More Responsive	
	First Born N = 8	Later Born N = 19	First Born N = 20	Later Born N = 8
Gesell—24 months				
M	102.6	96.3	106.9	102.5
S.D.	9.3	8.7	13.2	9.1
Stanford-Binet—5 Years				
M	98.2	99.2	110.6	110.4
S.D.	9.1	21.7	14.7	10.6
WISC-R—Full Scale—8 Years				
M	109.0	102.3	112.5	116.2
S.D.	13.5	16.1	14.1	17.9

caregiving acting alone nor in interaction were significant at 2 years ($p<.10$). At 5 years responsive caregiving was a significant main effect [F $(1,40) = 5.85$, $p<.05$] whereas at 8 years responsive caregiving just missed being significant at the conventional level, [F $(1,53) = 3.68$ $p<.06$]. At 5 and 8 years birth order was not significant itself nor did it enter into an interaction with responsive caregiving in terms of the child's cognitive development.

Table VI presents the data for maternal education and responsive caregiving. Mothers with 12 years or less of schooling were considered less educated whereas those with more than a high school education composed the more educated group. Although mothers who were more responsive were more educated there were a number of less educated mothers who were able to establish and maintain a responsive social environment for their children (39%). Conversely, there were some educated mothers who were unable to establish and maintain a responsive environment (37%). Responsive caregiving was significant as a main effect at each age period

TABLE VI

Cognitive Development Scores Related to Responsive Caregiving and Maternal Education

| | Less Responsive | | More Responsive | |
	Less Educated N = 17	More Educated N = 10	Less Educated N = 11	More Educated N = 17
Gesell—24 Months				
M	98.7	98.3	103.2	107.2
S.D.	8.7	10.4	10.5	13.1
Stanford-Binet—5 Years				
M	98.8	99.1	104.1	113.8
S.D.	19.0	17.4	14.2	12
WISC-R—Full Scale—8 Years				
M	105.1	103.0	108.1	117.1
S.D.	16.5	14.0	15.5	14.1

and maternal education was got significant [2 years $F (1,51) = 5.35$, p<.05; 5 years $F (1,49) = 4.53$, p<.05; 8 years $F (1,51) = 4.15$, p<.05]. The analyses suggest that it is good caregiving, regardless of mother's education, that is advantageous for the child's cognitive development.

Table VII presents the data for social class and responsive caregiving. The Hollingshead 4 factor Index was used to divide the sample at the median into high and low social class. Documentation of specific social encounters between a mother and her child indicated that at two years the responsivity of the mother, not social class, was associated with cognitive competence. The children of more responsive mothers scored higher on the Gesell Developmental Schedules at 24 months, regardless of social class, $F (1,51) = 4.95$, p<.05. By 5 years the early responsivity was not as important as the overall social class, and it was social class that was significantly associated with cognitive scores $F (1,49) = 6.33$, p<.05. At 8 years neither social class nor responsive caregiving were

TABLE VII

Cognitive Development Scores Related to Responsive Caregiving and Social Class

	Less Responsive		More Responsive	
	Lower SES N = 17	Higher SES N = 10	Lower SES N = 9	Higher SES N = 19
Gesell—24 Months				
M	98.2	98.3	103.7	106.6
S.D.	9.3	9.5	12.0	12.4
Stanford-Binet—5 Years				
M	97.6	101.0	97.5	116.1
S.D.	19.2	17.2	14.1	8.6
WISC-R—Full Scale—8 Years				
M	104.8	103.5	102.8	118.7
S.D.	16.2	14.8	15.3	12.2

significant as main effects, but showed a significant interaction, F $(1,51) = 4.34$, $p < .05$. The highest scoring group, significantly different from all others, was that which received responsive caregiving in infancy and had families of above average social class. The group from families of above average social class who had not experienced responsive caregiving in infancy performed no differently than did children from lower class families.

DISCUSSION

Children born preterm who experienced more responsive social interactions from their primary caregiver during infancy showed higher intelligence test scores from age 2 through age 8. The association held regardless of the children's gestational age, birthweight, number of days of neonatal hospitalization, or number of obstetrical or perinatal complications. As we have reported in several previous publications, for these children who were born in 1972–1974 and survived free of sensory and motor handicaps, medical factors were unrelated to their intellectual outcome. Home environmental factors were as important to their cognitive development as for children born healthy at term and not at biological risk (Gottfried, 1984). Medical factors may play a more salient role in the development of infants who survive in the 1980's who experience a more severe neonatal course. Yet , we expect that even for those very low birthweight infants, home environmental factors will be as important as within our study.

Although preterm infants are more difficult to care for and their parents are more stressed than are healthy infant—parent dyads, there was much variability in the degree to which the mother-infant dyad engaged in responsive interactions. Many of the dyads were able to compensate for their difficulties and to work out satisfying social interactions. Our findings are consistent with the contention that it is the relationship within the dyad that matters, not the degree of individual competence of either member of the dyad (Ainsworth, 1978; Goldberg, 1983). By conducting multiple cross-time home observations, we were able to make a stable and objective superordinate score that took into account the quality of the social interactions the child experienced from the caregiver across various time periods during infancy. It was not the ability to achieve responsiveness at one observation that mattered, but the ability to maintain responsiveness across time that was relevant to the child's later intellectual performance. Approximately half of the dyads maintained stable interactional patterns, either very responsive or very unresponsive, whereas half of the dyads shifted. It was the cumulative nature of the child's experience, not a single time period, that was significant.

The social experiences within the home were influenced by the ecology of the family (Bronfenbrenner, 1979). A number of factors influenced the degree to which the primary caregiver was responsive to her infant in social interactions. The findings give insights regarding potential mechanisms within the context of the family which regulate the social experiences in the home available to infants and to toddlers. A higher percentage of mothers engaged in responsive social interactions with their first-born infant, who was also the only young child in the home, than they did with their later born infant. Similarly, more mothers with education past high school provided responsive social experiences to their infant than did mothers who had either not graduated high school or had only high school education. Further, a greater number of mothers from the middle or upper class provided their infant with responsive social interactions than did lower class women. Despite those relationships, however, there was a tremendous diversity within social environments. Within every group, some infants experienced very responsive social interactions and some did not.

Thus, although global variables such as birth order and maternal education were linked to the responsiveness of the caregiver, when we looked within birth order and education groups we could see that there was no direct link between the global factors and cognitive development independent of the responsiveness of the caregiver. Our findings, consistent with Wachs and Gruen (1982), showed that significant variance was associated more with directly measured proximal environmental parameters, such as responsiveness of social interactions, than with global distal variables of parity and maternal education.

The covariation of social class and responsive social interaction revealed a more complex pattern. Infants from the middle class tended to receive more responsive social experience and those who did were more developmentally advanced by age 2. So were infants from the lower class who were treated more responsively. For that age, the social status of the family was less important than the relationship to the caregiver. By age 5, however, children from the lower class who had been treated more responsively in infancy no longer had a cognitive advantage, whereas the middle class children with similar early experience maintained their high level of intellectual competence. By age 8, neither the proximal events of early social experience nor the distal measure of family social status were linked directly to children's cognitive performance. By age 8, being reared in higher social class homes was insufficient, by itself, to produce highly intellectually achieving children. Good relationships with the mother during infancy were also insufficient to produce highly achieving school age children. Instead, both factors, an advantaged social class background and an advantaged relationship with the mother during infancy, were necessary to produce highly competent children.

The fact that both variables needed to be considered does not diminish the importance of responsive caregiving. We suggest the association between responsive caregiving and intellectual competence is not specific to experiences in infancy but is due to the continuity with later experience. If the association depends on a continuing responsive social environment then the link will be attenuated by the degree to which the environment is unstable. Parent-child relationships tend to be more unstable within the lower class than within the middle class (Egeland & Farber, 1984). Therefore, the association between responsive caregiving and intellectual competence will be stronger in the middle class than in the lower class, as we have found. Early experience does not act as an inoculation but only as a preview of a continuing process.

There are important implications for intervention programs. Regardless of position in the family, maternal education, and even social class, children's intellectual performance at school age can be enhanced if their parents can be helped to provide and maintain a more responsive social environment. Such environments would act as a protective factor in children's development, even children at biological risk.

References

Ainsworth, M.D.S., Blehar, M.C., Waters, E. & Walls, S. (Eds.) (1978). *Patterns of attachment*, Hillsdale, N.J.: Erlbaum.

Beckwith, L. & Cohen, S.E. (1984). Home environment and cognitive competence in preterm children in the first five years. In: A.W. Gottfried (Ed.), *Home environment and early mental development*, New York: Academic Press.

Bradley, R. & Caldwell, B. (1976). Early home environment and changes in mental test performance from 6 to 36 months, *Development Psychology*, **12**, 93–97.

Bronfenbrenner, U. (1979). *The ecology of human development*, Cambridge, MA: Harvard University Press 1979.

Clarke-Stewart, K.A. (1973). Interactions between mothers and their young children: Characteristics and consequences, *Monographs of the Society for Research in Child Development*, **38** (6–7, Serial No. 153).

Cohen, S.E. & Parmelee, A.H. (1983) Prediction of five year Stanford-Binet Scores in preterm infants, *Child Development*, **54**, 1242–53.

Cohen, S.E., Parmelee, A.H., Sigman, M., & Beckwith, L. (in press). Cognitive development of preterm infants: Birth to 8 years, *Journal of Developmental Behavioral Pediatrics*.

Davies, P.A. (1984). Follow-up of low birthweight children, *Archives of Diseases in Childhood*, **59**, 794–97.

Deutsch, C.P. (1973). Social class and child development. In: B.M. Caldwell & H.N. Ricciuti (Eds.), *Review of child development research* (Vol. 3), Chicago: University of Chicago Press.

Egeland, B. & Farber, E.A. (1984). Infant-mother attachment: Factors related to its development and changes over time. *Child Development*, **55**, 753–71.

Goldberg, S. & DiVitto, B.A. (Eds.) (1983). *Born too soon: Preterm birth and early development*, New York: W.H. Freeman & Co.

Gottfried, A.W. (Ed.) (1984). *Home environment and early cognitive development: Longitudinal research*, Orlando, Florida: Academic Press.

Kopp, C.B. (1983). Risk factors in development. In: M. Haith & J. Campos (Eds.), *Infancy and the biology of development*, Vol. II—from P. Mussen (Ed.), *Manual of child psychology*, New York: John Wiley & Sons.

Minde, K. (1980). Bonding of parents to premature infants: Theory and practice. In P.M. Taylor (Ed.), *Monographs in neonatology series*, New York: Grune & Stratton.

Moore, T. (1968). Language and intelligence: A longitudinal study of the first eight years (Part 2): Environmental correlates of mental growth, *Human Development*, **11**, 1–24.

Scarr, S. (Ed.) (1981). *Race, social class, and individual differences in IQ*, Hillsdale N.J.: Erlbaum.

Wachs, T.D. & Gruen, G.E. (Eds.) (1982). *Early experience and human development*, New York: Plenum.

Helping parents with preterm infants: Field test of a protocol[1]

KATHRYN E. BARNARD, MARY A. HAMMOND, GEORGINA
A. SUMNER, REBECCA KANG, NIA JOHNSON-CROWLEY,
CHARLENE SNYDER, ANITA SPIETZ, SUSAN BLACKBURN,
PATRICIA BRANDT, and DIANE MAGYARY

INTRODUCTION

Follow-up of the preterm and low birth weight infant is a particularly critical public health need. While recent evidence shows that the survival rate of premature infants continues to improve and the majority of preterm infants show normal developmental progress, the fact remains that many preterm infants do demonstrate developmental problems in later years. Sameroff (1981) recently summarized the two main conclusions that result from longitudinal studies of premature infants: first, that an estimated 20-50% of these children have later problems, and second, that the variables with the most power in predicting later outcomes are measures of the child's environment.

Many studies indicate that while the parent of a preterm infant may try harder in the beginning to stimulate and encourage the infant's development, preterm infants are less responsive to the parent (Beckwith & Cohen, 1980; Brown & Bakeman, 1979; Divitto & Goldberg, 1979; Field, 1977, 1980; Goldberg, Brachfeld, & Divitto, 1980). Likewise, over time the parent tends to become less responsive. We have found that during the latter half of the infant's first year a different interactive pattern emerges between a mother and her preterm infant. Based on the Premature Infant Refocus project data (Barnard, Bee & Hammond, 1984), the four and eight month mother-infant interactions were characterized by

[1]Supported by Maternal and Child Health Training, Grant No. MCH-009035, Bureau of Health Care and Delivery Assistance, Health Resources and Service Administration, Public Health Service, Department of Health and Human Services.

contrasting patterns. Four-month interactions were characterized by intense maternal involvement and limited infant responsiveness; eight month interactions in contrast were characterized by a less attentive and involved mother and a more alert and responsive infant. By two years of age we found that mothers of preterm infants provided less stimulation in the home environment than did mothers of term infants.

Recently Beckwith & Cohen (1983) presented data from the UCLA follow-up study of premature infants that confirm the phenomena of parent burnout during the first year of life. They showed that the level of maternal responsiveness changes over time and is highly related to the infant's condition. Infants with more health problems and prematurity had mothers who over time became less responsive. These findings on the interactive process raise questions about the disadvantage the parent-infant dyad may have in establishing attachment bonds. There is a need for continued study about parent-preterm infant interaction and for testing whether programs of preventive intervention can, in fact, prevent the decreased involvement and responsiveness of the parent during the first year of life (Magyary, 1983).

In studies comparing preterm and term infants, the results indicate that the premature infant has a decreased level of behavioral responsiveness and less organization of sleep-wake activity (Telzrow, Kang, Mitchell, *et al.*, 1982; Kang & Barnard, 1979; Barnard, 1980). Therefore, we have the situation where the infant in the early months provides less clear cues and less feedback to the caregiver and the caregiver over time, without this level of responsiveness and organization, becomes disorganized in the caregiving process and less involved.

Recently we have been involved in two major studies testing nursing intervention protocols with high risk families (Barnard, Booth, Mitchell, & Telzrow, 1983; Barnard, Bee, Booth, Magyary, Mitchell, & Sumner, 1982). The first of these studies, Models of Newborn Nursing Care, tested three models of nursing care to socially and medically risked infants and their families and demonstrated that with nursing intervention during the first three months of life, parent-child interaction did improve over the first two years.

Analysis comparing preterm and term infants from the Models of Newborn Nursing Care study revealed that the preterm infants and mothers in this nursing intervention study fared better than our previously reported comparisons of preterm and term infants without nursing follow-up (Barnard, Bee & Hammond, 1984). For this analysis, infants who were preterm (N = 10) and met the qualification to be in the study, which were complication of the pregnancy and social risk, were compared with term infants (N = 43) who also met the qualifications for the study but who had no other infant or family complications. The preterm infants had a higher pregnancy medical risk score and the nurses spent almost double the amount of time in follow-up during the first 3 months (472 versus 285 minutes). At 3 months on the Bayley Scales of Infant Development there were no preterm versus term differences. There were differences in the mother-infant interaction; preterm infants were less responsive during both the feeding and teaching observations. The mothers of preterms at 3 months were observed as having less desirable interaction in the feeding observation; and in observations on the HOME Inventory they scored lower on the mother's emotional and verbal responsivity and on maternal involvement. At the 10-month evaluation there were no parent-infant interaction differences. A surprising finding was that the preterm infants scored higher than the term infants on the Bayley Psychomotor Index. These results suggest that the nursing intervention helped sustain and even improve the parents' interaction and stimulation over the first year.

These findings with premature infants from the Models of Newborn Nursing Care project are supported by the work of Ross (1984) who reported a home intervention program for low income premature infants. The intervention consisted of public health nurse visits to the family to provide emotional support, instruction on the care and development of premature infants and a physical examination. Also, a pediatric therapist visited monthly to advise parents about feeding, handling, and stimulation. Each infant receiving intervention was matched to another infant from the same neonatal intensive care unit based on birth weight, social class, ethnicity, degree of parinatal illness and degree of neurological abnormality. The intervention and control groups were compared at one year of age post-term on the Bayley Scales of Infant Development, the Toddler Temperament Scale, the HOME, and an index of maternal attitudes toward childrearing. The results showed that infants in the home intervention group had significantly higher scores on the Bayley Mental Scales and on the HOME inventory. They did not differ on psychomotor ability or the maternal rating of temperament or maternal attitudes.

A few other intervention studies with preterm infants have been primarily mother-oriented, with the aim of influencing infant development by focusing on maternal attitudes and on caregiving and interaction skills. Bromwich and Parmelee (1979) in a center-based program for preterm infants and their families of varying social backgrounds, reported positive effects on the interactions and social skills of premature infants. In a home-based intervention program for teenage mothers of premature infants, Field, Widmayer, Stringer, *et al.* (1980) found higher ratings for both the mothers and the infants on face-to-face interactions at 4 months for the intervention group; at 8 months, the infants in the intervention group received higher Bayley mental scores and higher HOME scores.

Based on the documented vulnerabilities of premature infants and their parents and the apparent success of some parent-oriented intervention programs, the present program, Nursing Systems Toward Effective Parenting-Premature (NSTEP-P), was developed in order to address the need expressed by public health nurses for guidance in their follow-up of families of premature infants. From our extensive contact with public health nurses throughout the country, we found a need to have nurses aware of new findings to help them tailor nursing care to assist parents in understanding the preterm infant's less responsive behavior and in helping the parents deal with their heightened anxiety about the infant.

The nursing protocol we developed was based on studies of preterms, parenting, and the ecology of infants and families previously mentioned. The protocol was designed to complement a health agency's existing strategy. The NSTEP-P protocol was designed to assist the nurse in focusing on the particular problem of parenting a less mature, less well-organized, and less responsive infant. The expected benefit of the protocol was nurse satisfaction in providing care and increasingly optimal parenting of the infant. The basic content and format of the protocols are outlined in Table I.

These protocols were tested on 76 mothers and their infants. The nurses using the protocols were trained by our research team through a training grant provided by the Maternal and Child Health Division, Bureau of Health Care and Delivery Assistance (Grant Number MCH-009035).

FIELD TRIALS: METHOD

Subjects

The subjects in the field trials were 76 mothers and their premature or low birth weight infants. The criterion for entry into the program was birth weight under 2500 grams or less than 37 weeks gestational age. Each of the 23 nurses followed one to five families selected from their regular caseload. Thirty of the families were located in San Jose, California; 18 in Seattle, Washington; 10 in Chicago, Illinois; 7 in Red Bank, New Jersey; 6 Vancouver, Washington; and 5 in Anchorage, Alaska.

Procedure

Each nurse made a maximum of eight contacts (home visits) to the families from their caseloads who consented to participate in the NSTEP-P field trials. The first contact was scheduled to occur at approximately 1 week post-discharge or approximately 37 weeks conceptional age. The other visits were scheduled to occur at 38,

TABLE I
Issues and Specific Content Included in Protocols at Each Contact

Contact	1	2	3	4	5	6	7	8
Gestational Age	37	38	40	44	48	52	56	60
ISSUE	definition of state	sleep pattern	sleep pattern	sleep pattern	organization of sleep patterns	sleep pattern	organization of sleep patterns	sleep patterns
STATE REGULATION	modulation of state	massage	massage crying	massage crying sucking	massage			
BEHAVIORAL RESPONSIVENESS	behavior abilities / mother observation	interaction: eye contact: motor actions / mother observation	interaction: feeding concepts / mother observation	interaction: feeding observation / mother observation	interaction: feeding observation / home environment / teaching loop / mother observation	interaction: teaching observation / mother observation stimulation	interaction: home environment / mother observation stimulation	interaction: feeding observation / teaching observation / mother observation stimulation
HEALTH CONCERNS	nutrition temperature	nutrition illness safety	nutrition health monitor growth measures	nutrition health monitor	nutrition health monitor growth measures	nutrition health monitor	nutrition health monitor	nutrition health monitor growth measures developmental assessment
FAMILY AND COMMUNITY RESOURCES	demographics / support: appraisal	problem solving family survey support survey	problem solving community resources	problem solving community resources	problem solving	problem solving family response	problem solving	update on demographics family survey support survey

40, 44, 52, 56, and 50 weeks conceptional age. The visits were of varying lengths. The nurses followed a specific protocol for each of the visits. At each contact, the instruments which were to be used for the evaluation of the field trials were completed and sent to the NSTEP-P office at the University of Washington.

Instruments

Protocol Checklists were completed by the nurses at each contact to document the extent to which the nurses implemented the NSTEP-P protocols. These consisted of lists of the nursing activities that were to be carried out at each contact as part of the NSTEP-P protocol. The number of items in each protocol ranged from 15 to 30. The score derived from these checklists was the percentage of protocol items completed at each contact.

Instruments used to obtain family and infant data fell into three main categories: parent ecology, infant characteristics, and mother-infant interaction and stimulation.

Three instruments were used to obtain data on parent ecology. The Personal Resources Questionnaire-Part II (PRQ), developed by Brandt and Weinert (1982), is a self-report instrument designed to assess qualities of a person's social network. The PRQ's 25 item, 7-point scale provides an attitudinal estimate of the five relational functions of support defined by Weiss (1979): intimacy, worth, opportunity for nurturance, social integration, and the availability of informational, emotional, and material help. The authors reported content and face validity, modest predictive validity with dyadic satisfaction and family functioning, and an internal consistency (Cronbach's alpha) of .89. The perceived social support score derived from this questionnaire is the sum of the responses to the 25 items. This measure was obtained at the first and last contacts.

The Feetham Family Functioning Survey (FFFS), developed by Roberts and Feetham (1982), was designed to measure three areas of family function: relationship between the family and broader social units, relationships between the family and subsytems including the division of labor, and relationships between the family and each individual. The FFFS consists of 25 items, is designed to be self-administered, and takes approximately 10 minutes to complete. Each item is rated on three 7-point scales: how much is there now, how much should there be, and how important is this to me. The measure of each scale is the sum of the scores across items. A fourth indirect measure, the family function discrepant score, is derived as the absolute difference between "how much is there now" and "how much should there be." The authors reported an internal consistency (Cronbach's alpha) of .81 for the discrepant score. Test-retest reliability was .85 over a two-week period. Concurrent validity was established through significant correlations with the Family Functioning Index (Pless & Satterwhite, 1973). The measure used in the present analyses was the family function discrepant score computed as the sum of the discrepant scores across the 25 items. This measure was obtained at the first and last contacts.

Other parent ecology measures were derived from the Demographic Interviews developed by the NSTEP-P staff. The demographic measures obtained at the first contact included age, education, occupation, work status, and race of the mothers and fathers, and marital stauts, family income, source of income, and family size. Family social status was computed using Hollingshead's (1975) four-factor index of social status. Demographic measures obtained at the last contact included family size, marital status, mother's work status, and source of family income: these measures were used to analyze changes in demographic characteristics over time.

Three instruments were used to obtain data on infant characteristics. The Referral Information form, developed by the NSTEP-P staff was used to record data about the infant's characteristics at birth and during the hospital stay. These measures included gestational age and weight at birth and at discharge; length and head circumference at birth; and Apgar score at five minutes. A checklist of 10 risk factors was also completed based on the Postanal Complications Scale developed by Parmelee and Littman (1974).

The summary of Growth and Sleep-Wake Measures form was developed by the NSTEP-P staff to record weight, length, and head circumference at Contacts 1, 3, 5, and 8. Sleep-wake measures were also recorded at Contacts 3, 6, and 8. These sleep-wake measures were derived from the Nursing Child Assessment Sleep-Activity Records (NCASA) completed by the mothers. The sleep-wake measures included the amount of infant sleep time during the day and the amount of infant awake time during the day.

The Denver Prescreening Developmental Questionnaire (PDQ) was used at the last contact to screen the infants for developmental problems. Developed by Frankenburg, van Doorninck, Liddell, and Dick (1976), the PDQ was designed to identify those children who require a more thorough screening with the Denver Developmental Screening Test (DDST). Children positive on the DDST would then be referred for diagnostic assessment. The PDQ consists of ten age-appropriate questions at age levels ranging from 3 months to 6 years, and can be completed by parents or professionals. The score is the number of passes out of the ten age-appropriate items. In the normative sample of 1,141 children, the predictive value of a referral based on 8 or fewer passes is 23.3%. This value was increased to 46.2% for a referral based on 6 or fewer passes. In the present study, the nurses completed the PDQ based on their observations or on parent report for behaviors that the nurses had not observed.

Three instruments were used to assess mother-infant interaction and stimulation. Mother-infant interaction during feeding was assessed at Contacts 4, 5, and 8 using the Nursing Child Assessment Feeding Scale (NCAFS). This scale was developed by the investigators from an earlier rating system used in the Nursing Child Assessment (NCA) Project (Barnard & Eyres, 1979). The scale is composed of a set of 76 binary (yes/no) items describing a mother's and infant's activities during a normal feeding interaction. The items are arranged into six subscales, following Barnard's (1978) conceptualization of adaptive behaviors: infant's clarity of cues and responsiveness to caregiver, and mother's sensitivity to cues, alleviation of distress, cognitive growth fostering, and social-emotional growth fostering. Internal consistency coefficients

(Cronbach's alpha) are .83 and .73 for the mother's and infant's total scores, respectively. These scales have been shown to differentiate between the interactions of mothers of preterm infants and mothers of term infants (Barnard & Bee, 1982), and between mothers of failure-to-thrive infants and those with normally developing infants (Lobo, Barnard, & Cooms, 1982). Interrater reliability of at least 85% was achieved by each of the NSTEP-P nurses.

The Nursing Child Assessment Teaching Scale (NCATS) consists of 73 binary (yes/no) items which describe the interaction while the mother is teaching the child a simple task. The six subscales fall into the same categories as the NCAFS, although the items are specific to the teaching situation. Internal consistency estimates (Cronbach's alpha) for subscales of this instrument range from .44 to .84, and are highest for the total scores. Predictive validity studies with a small group of infants (N = 22) have shown sizeable (but not statistically significant) relationships between the NCATS scores and 4-year Stanford-Binet IQ's (r = .44 to .58) and between the NCATS scores and the HOME Inventory (r = .44 to .67). Interrater reliability of at least 85% was achieved by the NSTEP-P nurses prior to the program. The NCATS was used at Contacts 6 and 8.

The Home Observation for Measurement of the Environment (HOME) was administered at Contacts 5 and 7. This 45-item binary checklist was developed by Caldwell & Bradley (1978) and measures the amount and kind of social and cognitive stimulation available to the infant in the home. It is administered using a combination of interview and observation. Scores derived from the HOME include a total score and six subscale scores: emotional and verbal responsivity of the mother, avoidance of restriction and punishment, organization of the physical and temporal environment, provision of appropriate play materials, maternal involvement with child, and opportunities for variety in daily stimulation. The HOME has been found to be a potent predictor of later cognitive skills (Bradley & Caldwell, 1976; Bee, Barnard, Eyres, et al., 1982). All NSTEP-P nurses achieved at least 85% interrater reliability with this instrument prior to the program.

Mother's Evaluation

The Mother's Evaluation form was devised by the NSTEP-P staff to obtain feedback from the mothers about how they felt about the program. The first part of this form involved ratings on 5-point scales on the amount and frequency of help from the nurse in thirteen areas. Sample questions include: "How much did the nurse help you with the special concerns and/or problems of having a premature baby?" and "How often did the nurse provide information you needed for yourself or for your baby?". These ratings were averaged to form an overall index of the mother's perceived help from the program. The second part of this form included two questions relating to the frequency and length of the nurse's visits.

RESULTS

Analyses of the data from the field trials focused on the objective of the program: optimal parenting of the premature infant. The expectation was that measures of parent ecology, infant characteristics, and mother-infant interactions would improve or at least not deteriorate over time. Repeated measures analyses of variance or paired t-tests were used for all measures assessed at two or more timepoints to analyze such changes over time. In addition, family and infant measures were compared with normative samples, when available.

Since many of the analyses required complete data at two or more timepoints, missing data at any one timepoint could considerably reduce the number of cases included in the analyses of changes over time. For various reasons which will be discussed later, one or more instruments were not completed for approximately one-third of the cases. This was not a serious problem since at least 50 cases were included in all the analyses of changes over time. The number of home visits actually made at Contacts 1 and 2 was 76, 72 visits were made at Contact 3, 75 at Contact 4, 73 at Contact 5, 71 at Contact 6, 70 at Contact 7, and 67 at Contact 8.

The Sample

Descriptive statistics for the hospital referral information for the infants are shown in Table II. The mean gestational age at birth was 32.0 weeks (range = 24-37). The mean birth weight was

TABLE II

Referral Information

Referral Information	M	SD	N	Percent
Gestational age (weeks)				
at birth	32.0	2.8	74	—
at discharge	36.0	1.9	74	—
Weight (grams)				
at birth	1675.7	502.9	75	—
at discharge	2242.3	431.9	67	—
Length at birth (centimeters)	41.6	4.6	61	—
OFC at birth (centimeters)	29.0	2.7	36	—
Apgar at 5 minutes	7.8	1.1	57	—
Number of risk factors	3.7	2.2	74	—
Sex				
Female	—	—	36	48.6
Male	—	—	38	51.4
Unreported	—	—	2	—
Parity				
0 (adopted)	—	—	1	1.4
1	—	—	42	58.3
2	—	—	16	22.2
3-5	—	—	13	18.1
Unreported	—	—	4	—
Risk Factors				
Respiratory distress	—	—	48	70.6
Positive or suspected infection			29	42.6
Ventilatory assistance	—	—	40	58.8
Noninfectious illness or anomaly	—	—	16	23.5
Metabolic disturbance	—	—	17	25.0
Convulsion	—	—	0	0.0
Hyperbilirubinemia or exchange transfusion	—	—	49	72.1
Temperature disturbance	—	—	29	42.6
Not feeding within 48 hours	—	—	44	64.7
Surgery	—	—	4	5.9
Unreported	—	—	8	—

1675.7 grams (range = 760-2729); 41.3% of the infants weighed 1500 grams or less at birth. The mean Apgar score at 5 minutes was 7.8 (range = 5-9) and the mean risk score was 3.7 (range = 0-8) out of a possible 10 risk factors. The most frequent risk factors were hyperbilirubinemia or exchange transfusion (72.1%), respiratory distress (70.6%), not feeding within 48 hours (64.7%), and ventilatory assistance (58.8%). The infants were discharged from the hospital at a mean gestational age of 36.0 weeks (range = 33-43.9) and a mean weight of 2242.3 grams (range = 1588-5103). Slightly more than half of the infants were males (51.4%).

Demographic characteristics of the mothers and fathers are shown in Table III. The mothers had a mean age of 26.9 years (range = 18-44) and mean of 13.1 years of schooling (range = 8-19). The majority of the mothers were white (72.4%) and were married or living with a partner (81.6%). About half (51.2%) of the mothers had been working during their pregnancy but only 7.9% of the mothers were working at Contact 1. For over half of the mothers (58.3%), the study infant was their firstborn child.

The fathers had a mean age of 30.0 years (range = 17-52) and a mean of 14.1 years of schooling (range = 8-20). The majority of the fathers were employed (83%).

Average family size was 4.2 (range = 3-8). The median income was $15,000-$24,999 for the previous year; 19.7% depended on public assistance as their major source of income. The families were fairly evenly distributed among the social status categories (Hollingshead, 1975) based on occupational and educational levels of the mother and/or father. The majority (51.3%) fell into the two mid-level categories (skilled workers and minor professionals); 24.8% fell into the lower two social status categories (unskilled and semiskilled workers); and 20.3% fell into the highest category (major professionals).

Dropouts

The data presented in this report are from the 76 families who remained in the program at least through the fourth contact. The number of families originally enrolled in the program was 101.

TABLE III
Demographic Information

Demographic Information	M	SD	N	Percent
Mother's age (years)	26.9	5.6	76	—
Father's age (years)	30.9	6.7	58	—
Mother's education (years)	13.1	2.3	76	—
Father's education (years)	14.1	2.9	57	—
Number of people in household	4.2	1.3	76	—
Social status score	39.4	15.0	74	—
Mother's race				
White	—	—	55	72.4
Black, Asian, Hispanic, other	—	—	21	27.6
Father's race				
White	—	—	42	72.4
Black, Asian, Hispanic, other	—	—	16	27.6
Unreported	—	—	18	—
Marital status				
Married or living with partner	—	—	62	81.6
No spouse or partner	—	—	14	18.4
Mother's work status				
Not working	—	—	37	48.7
Worked during past 9 months	—	—	33	43.3
Working now	—	—	6	7.9
Father's work status				
Not working	—	—	6	10.2
Worked during past 9 months	—	—	4	6.8
Working now	—	—	49	83.1
Unreported	—	—	17	—
Income[a]				
Less than $7,500	—	—	13	20.6
$7,500—14,999	—	—	13	20.6
$15,000—24,999	—	—	14	22.2
$25,000—39,999	—	—	12	19.0
$40,000 or more	—	—	11	17.5
Unreported	—	—	13	—
Source of income				
Employment (self and/or spouse)	—	—	58	76.3
Public assistance	—	—	13	17.1
Parents, scholarships, other	—	—	5	6.6

[a]Median income = $15,000-$24,999

Twenty-five of these families (24.8%) dropped out of the program before the fourth contact. Most of these early dropouts were due to moving or returning to work. Another 6 families (5.9%) dropped out after the fourth contact. Most of these later dropouts were due to the same reasons, but a few chose not to continue because they felt the visits were no longer helpful. The data from those who dropped out before the fourth contact are not included in the present analyses.

Differences between the early dropouts ($N = 25$) and those who remained in the study ($N = 76$) were examined. In comparison to the infant characteristics shown in Table II for those who remained in the study, the dropouts had a significantly lower Apgar score at 5 minutes ($M = 6.8$), but did not differ significantly on gestational age, birth weight, length, OFC, or the number of risk factors.

While the infants who dropped out of the program were not very different from those who remained, there were several significant differences on the family demographic variables. Compared to the families who remained in the study (see Table III), the mothers who dropped out were significantly younger ($M = 22.5$ years) and had significantly less schooling ($M = 11.9$ year). The fathers in the families who dropped out were also significantly younger ($M = 26.1$ years) and had significantly less schooling ($M = 11.8$ years). The families who dropped out had significantly lower income levels (median $5,000–$9,999); 50% were on public assistance. Their social status scores were also significantly lower ($M = 27.5$), and tended to be in the semi-skilled workers category. There were no significant differences between the early dropouts and those who remained, on mother's race, father's race, or marital status.

Protocol Implementation

The percentage of protocol items completed, derived from the Protocol Checklists, was used to analyze the degree to which the nurses implemented the NSTEP-P protocols. (The total number of items in each protocol ranged from 15 to 30.) In general, the nurses completed a high percentage of items in each of the eight protocols. The mean percentage of items completed for each protocol ranged from 90.6 to 97.6%. The standard deviations ranged from about 9 to 14%.

The concept of state modulation was introduced to 100% of the mothers at Contact 1 and NCASA records were given to 95–99% of the mothers at the first five contacts. The NCASA or 24-hour recall of the infant's sleep-wake patterns were discussed with 92–99% of the mothers at Contacts 2–5.

The concept of behavioral responsiveness was introduced at Contact 1 to 100% of the mothers, although visual and auditory responsiveness was demonstrated with only 75% of the infants, presumably because the infants were asleep. The Mother's Observation Record (MOR) was given to 92–98% of the mothers in each of the first seven contacts, and the MOR's that were completed by the mothers were reviewed in 88–93% of the succeeding contacts. Massage was introduced to 98% of the mothers in Contact 2. Because some of the mothers chose not to use the massage techniques, massage was reviewed for only 84–90% of the mothers in the next three contacts. Play activities were introduced to 96% of the mothers in Contact 6 and Play was discussed with 97–99% of the mothers in the next two contacts. Feeding guidelines were discussed with 98% of the mothers at Contact 3 and feeding observations were completed with 88–93% of the mothers and infants at Contact 4, 5, and 8. The teaching loop was introduced to 100% of the mothers at Contact 5, and teaching observations were completed with 90–92% of the mothers and infants at Contacts 6 and 8. The HOME was completed with 99% of the families at Contacts 5 and 7.

In the area of health related concerns, nutrition, feeding, and growth was discussed with 99–100% of the mothers at each of the eight contacts. Physical environment and safety were discussed with 84–96% of the mothers at the first three contacts, signs and symptoms of illness were discussed with 98% of the mothers at the Contact 2, and health care maintenance was dicussed with 99–100% of the mothers in Contacts 4–8.

In the area of family and community resources, the problem solving form was the least utilized. Because either the nurse or the mother did not feel it was necessary, problem solving was discussed with only 88% of the mothers at Contact 2. Problem solving forms were given to 75–87% of the mothers at Contact 2, 5, and 6, and were completed by and reviewed with only 60–79% of the mothers in succeeding contacts. Information on community resources was discussed with 90% of the mothers in Contact 4 and coping strategies were discussed with 85–89% of the mothers in Contacts 5 and 6.

In the area of anticipatory guidance, the Parent Activities sheet was reviewed and given to 92–98% of the mothers in Contacts 1–7, and the activities from the previous contact were reviewed with 86–95% of the mothers in Contacts 2–8.

Family and Infant Evaluations

Parent Ecology.   Two measures of parent ecology were perceived social support and an index of family function. Other demographic measures were used to evaluate family stability. These measures were obtained at Contacts 1 and 8 and are shown in Table IV.

The measure of perceived social support was derived from the Personal Resources Questionnaire-Part II (PRQ). The score is the sum of the responses to 25 7-point scales related to perceived social support in the areas of intimacy, social integration, nurturance, worth, and assistance. The possible range of scores is 25-175; the higher the score, the greater amount of perceived social support. For this sample, the internal consistency (alpha coefficients) of the scale was .87 and .89 at Contacts 1 and 8, respectively.

For the 55 mothers who completed the PRQ at Contact 1 and Contact 8, the mean perceived social support scores were 140.8 and 142.2, respectively. A paired *t*-test between these scores at the two timepoints showed no significant difference between Contact 1 and Contact 8 on the amount of perceived social support. The correlation between these scores at the two timepoints was .76 (p<.01). These statistics suggest a high degree of stability over time on the amount of perceived social support.

Compared to other samples, the perceived social support score for the NSTEP-P sample is equivalent to the mean score of 140.5 (SD = 17.9) obtained by Lobo (1982) in a sample of 188 middle-

C

TABLE IV

Changes Over Time: Parent Ecology Measures

| Measure | Contact 1 | | Contact 8 | | | |
	M	SD	M	SD	t	N
Personal Resources Questionnaire—Part II						
Perceived Social support	140.8	17.1	142.2	17.9	−0.9	55
Feetham Family Functioning Survey						
Family function discrepant score	24.5	13.2	22.5	14.3	1.3	59
Demographic Interview						
Number of people in household	4.3	1.4	4.3	1.4	1.1	66

| Measure | Contact 1 | | Contact 8 | |
	N	Percent	N	Percent
Demographic Interview				
Marital status				
Married or living with partner	51	79.7	53	82.8
No spouse or partner	13	20.3	11	17.2
Mother's work status				
Working or in school	4	6.1	26	39.4
Not working	62	93.9	40	60.6
Source of income				
Employment (self and/or spouse)	50	76.9	50	76.9
Public assistance	15	23.1	15	23.1

class couples attending prenatal classes, and significantly higher than the mean score of 134.4 ($SD = 24.9$) obtained by Murtaugh (1982) in a sample of 77 low income mothers.

The measure derived from the Feetham Family Functioning Survey (FFFS) was the family function discrepant score. This score is the sum of the discrepant scores across the 25 items; the higher the score, the greater the discrepancy between "what is" and "what should be". The possible range for this score is 0–150. Because 9 of the 25 items apply only to respondents with partners, an adjusted score was computed for mothers without partners (adjusted score = average score on items answered × 25). For this sample, the internal consistency (alpha coefficients) of the family function discrepant score was .79 and .86, at Contacts 1 and 8, respectively.

For the 59 mothers who completed the FFFS at both contacts, there was a small non-significant decrease in the family function discrepant score from 24.5 at Contact 1 to 22.5 at Contact 8. The correlation between these scores at the two timepoints was .61 (p<.01). As with the social support measure, family function appears to be relatively stable over this time period for this sample. The mean family function discrepant scores for the NSTEP-P sample are equivalent to the mean of 24.2 ($SD = 11.1$) obtained by Thomas and Barnard (1986) in a sample of well-educated mothers of children with a mean age of 2.5 years.

The correlations between perceived social support and the family function discrepant score were −.34 (<.01) at Contact 1 and −.61 (p<.01) at Contact 8. These moderate correlations suggest that these two measures of parent ecology are tapping somewhat different constructs.

Other parent ecology variables which could be examined over time came from the Demographic Interviews at Contacts 1 and 8. The number of people in the household remained stable at a mean of 4.3 people at both contacts. There were few changes in marital status over time; only two of the 13 mothers who were not married or living with a partner at Contact 1 acquired a spouse or partner by Contact 8. The proportion of families on public assistance also remained stable over time. Only one of the 15 families who had been on public assistance became employed by Contact 8; and one family whose source of income was from employment at Contact 1 was on public assistance at Contact 8.

The mother's work status did change markedly over time; 37.1% of the mothers who had not been working at Contact 1 were working or in school at Contact 8. One of the four mothers who was working at Contact 1 was not working at Contact 8. These changes over time for marital status, source of income, and mother's work status could not be analyzed statistically because of the low number of cases in some cells.

Infant Characteristics. Growth measures taken at birth, and at Contacts 1, 3, 5, and 8 were analyzed with repeated measures analyses of variance which showed significant increases in weight, height, and head circumference across the five timepoints. Paired *t*-tests between successive timepoints showed significant increases between each successive timepoint for all three growth measures. The plots for weight were typical of those for premature infants as described by Gairdner and Pearson (1971).

Sleep-wake measures came from data at Contacts 3, 6, and 8. The two sleep-wake measures derived from the NCASA records completed by the mothers were amount of infant sleep time during the day and amount of infant awake time during the day. The "day" was defined as the period of time from when the mother got up in the morning to the time she went to sleep at night. The amount of infant sleep during the day ranged from a mean of 7.5 hours at Contact 3 to a mean of 4.1 hours at Contact 8. This overall decrease over time and decreases between each successive time point were statistically significant. Similarly and in a reciprocal manner, the amount of infant awake time during the day increased significantly over time from a mean of 6.0 hours at Contact 3 to a mean of 9.2 hours at Contact 8. Increases between each successive timepoint were also significant for the amount of awake time during the day.

The Denver Prescreening Developmental Questionnaire (PDQ), was given at Contact 8. The PDQ score was calculated as the number of items passed (out of ten items) at the infant's adjusted age level. Adjusted age was calculated as living age in weeks at Contact 8 minus the number of weeks the infant was born prior to 40 weeks gestation. This adjusted was then converted to months to calculate PDQ scores at the appropriate age levels of 4, 5, or 6 months adjusted age. The appropriate (adjusted) age levels on the PDQ were 4 months for 3.1% of the 65 infants who had PDQ data, 5 months for 50.8% of the infants, and 6 months for 46.2% of the infants. For two infants where Contact 8 occurred much later than the proposed schedule (8 and 10 months adjusted age), PDQ scores could not be calculated.

Six percent of the infants had 6 or fewer passes at their adjusted age level. According to the normative data (Frankenburg *et al.*, 1976), there is a 46.2% chance that these infants would not score in the normal range on the more thorough screening test, the Denver Developmental Screening Test (DDST), and then would require diagnostic assessment if they did not pass the DDST. Another 18.5% of the infants in the NSTEP-P sample scored 7 or 8 passes on the PDQ. The predictive value of these scores is 23.3% and they are classified as questionable since they may represent only temporary delays. Finally, 75.4% of the infants had nonsuspect (normal) scores of 9 or 10 passes. The percentage of infants in the NSTEP-P sample with suspect (abnormal) scores (6.2%) is roughly equivalent to the figure of 6.8% found in the Franken-burg's *et al.* (1976), sample of 1,141 children aged 3 months to 6 years.

Mother-Infant Interaction and Stimulation.   Scores from the Nursing Child Assessment Feeding Scale for 50 cases for whom feeding observations were completed at Contacts 4, 5, and 8 are given in Table V. Repeated measures analyses of variance showed significant increases over time on all the subscales and total scores except the mother's sensitivity to cues and response to distress.

Paired *t*-tests between each of the timepoints showed that the infant's responsiveness to the mother increased significantly between each successive contact, and clarity of cues increased significantly between Contacts 4 and 5 and remained stable between Contacts 5 and 8. The mother's scores on cognitive growth fostering increased significantly between Contacts 4 and 5 and then remained stable through Contact 8, and social-emotional growth fostering increased significantly from Contact 4 to Contact 8.

These scores from the feeding interaction for the NSTEP-P sample were compared to data from the NCAST normative sample of term infants at equivalent adjusted ages and at equivalent living ages. Differences between the two samples were analyzed using *t*-tests. For adjusted age comparisons, data from the normative sample at 1, 2, and 5 months of age were compared to the NSTEP-P sample at Contacts 4, 5, and 8, respectively. For living age comparisons, data from the normative sample at 3, 4, and 7 months were compared to the NSTEP-P sample at Contacts 4, 5 and 8, respectively. The number of cases in the NCAST normative

TABLE V

Changes Over Time: Nursing Child Assessment Feeding Scale

Subscales and Total Scores	Contact 4		Contact 5		Contact 8		F	Significant Contrasts
	M	SD	M	SD	M	SD		
Mother								
Sensitivity to cues	14.3	1.9	14.6	1.4	14.6[ab]	1.4	1.1	—
Response to distress	10.2	1.5	10.5	1.0	10.6[ab]	0.7	2.1	—
Social-emotional growth fostering	12.1	2.0	12.4	1.6	12.9[a]	1.5	5.3*	8>4
Cognitive growth fostering	6.3	2.5	7.2[a]	1.6	7.5	1.7	9.0**	8,5>4
Total mother score	43.1	6.6	44.7[ab]	4.5	45.6[ab]	3.7	7.9**	8,5>4
Infant								
Clarity of cues	12.4	1.7	13.0[a]	1.9	13.4[a]	1.8	5.8**	8,5>4
Responsiveness to mother	6.8[c]	2.3	7.9[a]	2.4	8.7	1.8	13.6**	8>5>4
Total infant score	19.2	3.6	20.8[a]	4.0	22.1[a]	3.4	11.9**	8>5>4
Total score	62.0	9.1	65.4[a]	7.7	67.5[a]	6.2	14.6**	8>5>4

NOTE. Data are tabled for 50 cases with scores at all three contacts.

[a]Significantly ($p<.05$) higher than norms at same adjusted age
[b]Significantly ($p<.05$) higher than norms at same living age
[c]Significantly ($p<.05$) lower than norms at same living age
*$p<.05$ **$p<.01$

sample ranged from 64 to 97; these data are cross-sectional.

In general, the infant's scores on the feeding interaction tended to be equivalent to both living age and adjusted age norms at Contact 4, except that the infant's responsiveness to mother was significantly lower than the living age norms. At Contact 5, the infant's scores tended to be equivalent to the living age norms and significantly higher than the adjusted age norms. And at Contact 8, the infant's clarity of cues and the total infant score were significantly higher than the adjusted age norms (see footnotes on Table V).

The mother's scores on the feeding interaction tended to be equivalent to both living age and adjusted age norms, at Contact 4. At Contact 5, only one of the mother's subscales (cognitive growth fostering) was significantly higher than the adjusted age norms, but the total mother score was significantly higher than both the living age and adjusted age norms. And at Contact 8, the total mother score was significantly higher than both norm groups, particularly due to higher scores on sensitivity to cues and response to distress. These comparisons for the mother's and infant's total feeding scores are illustrated in Figures 1 and 2.

Scores from the Nursing Child Assessment Teaching Scale for the 57 cases who had data at Contacts 6 and 8 are shown in Table VI. The only significant change over time was a singificant increase in the mother's cognitive growth fostering.

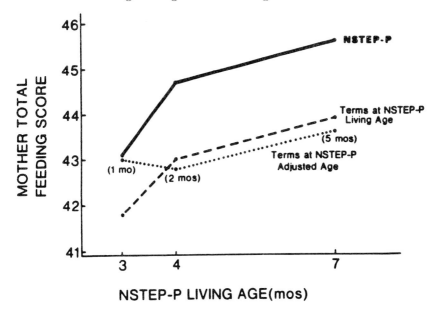

FIGURE 1 Mother's total feeding score for NSTEP-P sample compared to normative sample of term infants.

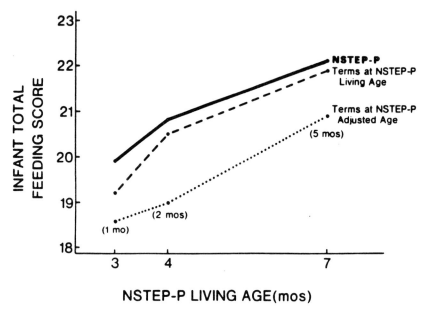

FIGURE 2 Infant's total feeding score for NSTEP-P sample compared to normative sample of term infants.

The teaching interaction data were also compared to the NCAST normative sample of term infants at 3 and 5 months for adjusted age comparisons and at 5 and 7 months for living age comparisons. A smaller normative sample size $(N = 33\text{-}38)$ was available for these comparisons. In general, the NSTEP-P infants and the mothers tended to be performing about the same as the normative sample on all subscales. The only significant difference was a significantly higher mean for the NSTEP-P sample on cognitive growth fostering at Contact 8 than the normative sample at the same adjusted age. Figures 3 and 4 illustrate these comparisons for the mother and infant total teaching scores.

Scores from the Home Observation for Measurement of the Environment (HOME) are shown in Table VII for 70 cases who had data at Contacts 5 and 7. Paired t-tests showed significant increases between the two timepoints on responsivity of mother,

TABLE VI

Changes Over Time: Nursing Child Assessment Teaching Scale

Subscales and Total Scores	Contact 6		Contact 8		
	M	SD	M	SD	t
Mother					
Sensitivity to cues	9.5	1.3	9.6	1.3	−0.6
Response to distress	10.4	1.3	10.5	0.9	−0.8
Social-emotional growth fostering	9.8	1.3	9.6	1.2	1.0
Cognitive growth fostering	12.6	3.5	13.6[a]	3.1	−2.3*
Total mother score	42.2	5.7	43.3	5.1	−1.6
Infant					
Clarity of cues	7.7	1.6	7.9	1.6	−1.0
Responsiveness to mother	7.4	3.2	7.2	3.3	0.5
Total infant score	15.1	4.3	15.1	4.5	−0.1
Total score	57.3	8.5	58.4	8.3	−1.2

NOTE: Data are tabled for 57 cases with scores at both contacts.
[a]Significantly ($p<.05$) higher than norms at same adjusted age
*$p<.05$

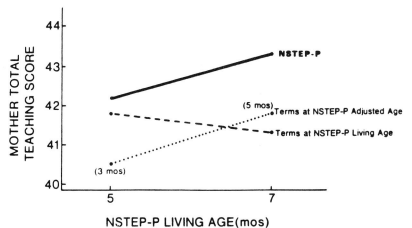

FIGURE 3   Mother's total teaching score for NSTEP-P sample compared to normative sample of term infants.

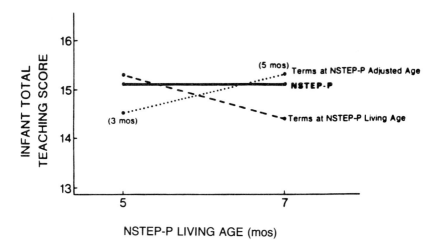

FIGURE 4   Infant's total teaching score for NSTEP-P sample compared to normative sample of term infants.

provision of appropriate play materials, opportunities for variety in daily stimulation, and on the total HOME score.

These NSTEP-P data were compared to data from the NCAST normative sample of term infants at 2 and 4 months for

TABLE VII

Changes Over Time: Home Observation for Measurement of the Environment

Subscales and Total Score	Contact 5		Contact 7		
	M	SD	M	SD	t
Responsivity of mother	9.9[a]	1.2	10.2[a]	1.2	2.5*
Avoidance of restriction	6.9	0.9	6.9	0.9	0.2
Organization of environment	5.3[a]	0.8	5.2	0.8	0.7
Play materials	6.0	2.0	6.7[b]	1.9	4.4**
Maternal involvement	5.4[a]	1.0	5.6[a]	0.9	1.5
Daily stimulation	2.8	1.1	3.1	1.1	2.5*
Total HOME Score	36.2[a]	4.5	37.6	4.2	5.00**

NOTE: Data are tabled for 70 cases with scores at both contacts.
[a]Significantly ($p < .05$) higher than norms at same adjusted age
[b]Significantly ($p < .05$) lower than norms at same living age
*$p < .05$ **$p < .01$

comparisons at the same adjusted age, and at 4 and 6 months for comparisons at the same living age. The normative sample size ranged from 99 to 116.

At Contact 5, the HOME scores for the NSTEP-P sample were not significantly different from those for the living age norms, but significantly higher than the adjusted age norms on responsivity to mother, organization of environment, maternal involvement, and the total HOME score. At Contact 7, the NSTEP-P scores continued to be equivalent to living age norms, except that they were significantly lower than living age norms on the play materials subscale. Comparisons with adjusted age norms at Contact 7 showed the NSTEP-P sample to be significantly higher on responsivity of mother and maternal involvement. These comparisons for the total HOME score are illustrated in Figure 5.

Mothers' Evaluation.   The mother's Evaluation form was completed by 50 mothers at the end of the program. The first part of this form involved ratings on 5-point scales of the amount and frequency of help from the nurse in thirteen areas. These ratings were averaged to form an overall index of the mother's perceived help from the

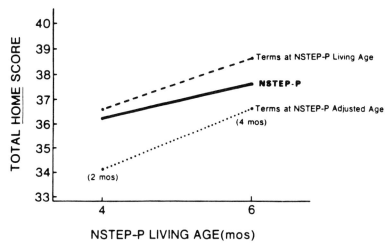

FIGURE 5   Total HOME score for NSTEP-P sample compared to normative sample of term infants.

program. This 13-item scale had an internal consistency (alpha coefficient) of .83. The mean overall score of the mother's perceived help from the program was 4.1, indicating "a good bit" and "frequent" help. The overall scores ranged from 2.3 to 5.0.

Predictive Relationships

A final question of interest is, how do the early characteristics of the infant and demographic/ecological characteristics of the mother relate to the "outcomes" for the infant and mother at the end of the program? To address this quetion, we have examined the correlations between selected measures of the infant and mother at referral and Contact 1, and selected "outcome" measures from Contacts 7 and 8. These correlations are shown in Table VIII.

Many of the birth characteristics of the infant related in expected ways to the outcome measures. For example, "healthier" infants at birth (higher birth weights, higher gestational ages, and lower risk scores) tended to be awake more hours of the day at Contact 8 than "less healthy" infants. In addition, males and infants with high birth weights tended to weigh more at Contact 8. Somewhat surprising is the positive relationship between gestational age at birth and the PDQ; even though the PDQ score is essentially adjusted for gestational age, the prematurity factor still appears to be influencing development. None of the birth characteristics of the infant were related to later feeding interaction scores. Surprisingly, infants with lower gestational ages and higher risk scores appear to be more responsive during the teaching situation. One explanation of this finding might be that the "healthier" infants at birth showed a normal decrease in responsiveness to the mother at this age (see pattern for normative sample of term infants between 5 and 7 months living age in Figure 4).

Another interesting relationship is that mothers who perceived the NSTEP-P program as more helpful, tended to be mothers of "less healthy" infants at birth (lower gestation ages, lower birth weights, and high risk scores). Although none of the mother's characteristics were related to her perceived help from the program, the nurses' ratings of the mother's progress were higher for

TABLE VIII
Correlations Between Early Mother and Infant Characteristics and Later Outcome Measures

	Outcome Measures (Contacts 7 and 8)												
	Nurse's Evaluation		Parent Ecology		Infant Characteristics			Mother-Infant Interaction and Stimulation					Mother's Evaluation
Early Measures (Contact 1)	Mother's progress	Infant's progress	Perceived social support	Family function discrepant score	Day hours awake	Weight	PDQ	Mother's feeding score	Intant's feeding score	Mother's teaching score	Infant's teaching score	Total home score	Perceived help from program
Infant													
Gestational age-birth	.02	.12	.15	−.18	.37**	.19	.27*	−.06	−.02	−.13	−.31**	.09	−.39**
Birth weight	.04	.15	.29*	−.21	.29*	.43**	.36**	.15	.14	.02	−.13	.25*	−.34**
Number of risk factors	−.13	−.26*	−.21	.05	−.27*	.02	−.14	.10	.13	.17	.28*	−.13	.24*
Sex (high = male)	−.05	−.10	−.22*	.13	−.11	.30**	−.11	.10	.10	.16	−.03	−.09	−.02
Mother													
Parity	−.12	.18	−.09	.24*	−.16	−.23*	−.38**	−.29*	−.15	−.11	−.07	.04	.13
Age	−.25*	−.11	−.05	−.11	−.16	.02	−.05	−.07	.04	.06	.25*	.09	.17
Education	−.04	−.17	−.04	−.12	−.11	.01	−.08	.20	−.01	.13	.16	.25*	−.21
Marital status (high = partner)	−.27	−.14	.20	−.21	−.10	.05	−.01	−.07	.02	.05	.14	.20*	−.16
Race (high = white)	.01	−.21*	.45**	−.22	−.05	.03	.02	.32**	.15	.24*	.06	.55**	−.13
Social status	−.02	−.17	.12	−.12	−.11	.15	−.10	.15	−.06	.18	.11	.42**	−.05
Perceived social support	.29*	.15	.76**	−.40**	.16	.06	−.14	.19	−.09	−.04	−.21	.30**	−.14
Family function discrepant score	−.25*	.07	−.44**	.61**	−.11	−.13	.03	−.02	.01	−.08	.09	−.20	.17

*p < .05 **p < .01

69

younger mothers and those without partners. Mothers with higher perceived social support and lower family function discrepant scores were also rated more highly on their progress. Infants who had higher progress ratings tended to be non-white and to have lower risk scores.

Several of the mother's characteristics related to the total HOME score in expected ways; mother's with higher HOME score tended to be more highly educated, married, white, and to have higher social status scores and higher perceived social support. The mother's feeding and teaching scores both tended to be higher for whites than for non-whites, but other demographic variables such as age and education (which are often found in other samples to be related to these scores), did not relate to the mother's feeding and teaching scores in this sample.

Parity showed some rather unexpected relationships with several of the outcome variables; mother's with more children tended to have higher family function discrepant scores, lower total feeding scores, and to have infants who weigh less and have poorer development at Contact 8. The possibility that these later two variables showed significant relationship with parity because of an underlying relationship between parity and birth weight was examined by running partial correlations. Using birth weight as a control variable, the partial correlations between parity and infant weight at Contact 8, and between parity and PDQ score, were still significant.

DISCUSSION

The results of the field trials support the main objectives of the NSTEP-P program: optimal parenting of the premature infant. The expectation was that measures of parent ecology, infant characteristics, and mother-infant interactions would improve or at least not deteriorate over time, and that these measures for the NSTEP-P sample would be comparable to data from normative samples of term infants.

In support of this objective, the parent ecology measures of perceived social support and the family function discrepant score remained stable over the eight contacts. Significant improvement in these parent ecology measures was not expected for this middle-class sample since their initial levels of support and family function tended to be high, therefore allowing little room for improvement. However, further analyses showed that mothers with high (above the sample mean) family function discrepant scores at the first contact, did show a significant decrease on this score over time. This finding suggests that the information provided to the mothers relating to family and community resources may have been more beneficial to mothers with high family disfunction. This suggests an area of the NSTEP-P protocols that could be modified depending on the needs of the individual mothers in the area of family and community resources. Indeed, we found that many of the nurses in this program did delete this section of the protocols when they felt that this information was not needed.

Also in support of this objective, the infants' growth progressed steadily over time, following the typical pattern for healthy premature infants, and leading to normal weight at approximately term age. Sleep-wake patterns also followed the predicted course, with significant increases in awake time during the year. And the infants' developmental levels at 5 months adjusted age approximated those of a normative sample, with only about 6% of the infants showing suspect scores on the screening test.

Results from the interactive observations also lend support to the study's objective. In the feeding interaction, significant increases in the infants "responsiveness and clarity of cues were accompanied by significant increases in the mother" social-emotional and cognitive growth fostering during the 16-week period between the first and last feeding observations. During the shorter 8-week period between the two teaching observations, significant increases were found only on the mother's cognitive growth fostering. However, for both feeding and teaching interactions, both the mothers and the infants were performing as well as, and in some cases better than, a normative sample of term infants at the same conceptional age. In the 8-week period between HOME observations, the mothers showed significant overall increases in the quality of the stimulation provided in the home environment, at levels equivalent to those found in a normative sample of term infants.

The data from the interactive observations, particularly during feeding, suggest the possibility of a specific treatment effect. While direct comparisons to non-intervention samples cannot be made, the data do suggest that the mothers and preterm infants in this program show a different developmental course in their interactions from those in non-intervention studies of mother-preterm interaction (see review by Magyary, 1984). In particular, the typical pattern found in early observations of interaction of a hyperattentive mother and an unresponsive infant are not seen in this sample; at 3 months living age, the mothers in this sample were performing at about the same level as mothers in a normative sample of term infants, and the infants were as responsive as term infants at the same conceptional age. By 4 months living age, the mothers appeared to be more attentive than mothers in the normative sample of term infants, but at the same time the infants were becoming more responsive. Finally, the tendency observed in non-intervention studies for mothers of preterm infants to gradually reduce their involvement with the infants during the second six months of life, is not seen in this sample. At least by 7 months living age, the mothers is this sample were not showing any evidence of maternal "burnout".

Emphasizing again that we cannot attribute the interaction patterns observed directly to the intervention, it can be noted that the findings appear to be a logical consequence of the specific training provided to the mothers. In the contacts prior to the first feeding observation, considerable emphasis was placed on teaching the mother an awareness of her infant's state changes and cues, and how to use the cues as a basis for providing an optimal interaction with her infant. Specific techniques were taught for arousing the infant in order to bring him to a more alert state for feeding and interacting. Behavioral responsiveness was discussed and demonstrated and the mothers kept observation records of how their infants responded in various situations. These principles were then applied specifically to the feeding situation. And finally, after the feeding observations, the mothers were given feedback and suggestions for improving the interaction. The results from the feeding observations suggest that providing the mothers with this kind of information and training may have promoted increased behavioral responsiveness on the part of the infant and increased the quality of the stimulation provided by the mother during the feeding interaction.

Such effects related to the specific intervention have been reported by Field *et al.* (1980) in their study of teenage, lower-class, black mothers, and their preterm infants. One of the training components in this program involved exercises designed to facilitate mother-infant interactions. At 4 months, both the teenage mothers and their preterm infants in the intervention group received more optimal face-to-face interactions ratings than did the control-group dyads. Similar effects were found by Fuhrmann (1984) in a control-intervention group study where mothers of preterm infants were given instruction on state related behaviors and state modulation prior to hospital discharge. The mothers in the intervention group were also given reading materials and kept detailed records of their infants' states prior to feeding for the first week after discharge. At 7 weeks living age, mothers and preterm infants in the intervention group both scored significantly higher on the Nursing Child Assessment Feeding Scale than the control group.

Our results on the teaching interactions and the HOME might also be cautiously interpreted as a logical consequence of the specific information provided to the mothers in the program. Prior to the first teaching observations, the principles of the teaching loop were discussed. These principles of alerting the infant, providing appropriate instructions, allowing the infant to perform, and providing feedback to the infant, related specifically to the cognitive growth fostering subscale which showed a significant increase over time. Prior to the first HOME observation, the nurse extended the principles of interaction to the overall organization of the infant's environment on a daily basis and discussed age appropriate play activities. These aspects of the protocol relate specifically to the HOME subscales which showed increases over time—variety in daily stimulation and provision of appropriate play materials.

Although interpretation of the present findings must be cautious, the present results show, at the very least, that the mothers and infants in this nursing intervention program showed stable or improving patterns of interaction over the first seven months of life. Further investigation is needed to determine whether these findings can be attributed to the intervention and whether the intervention has sustained impact on these infants and their families.

References

Barnard, K.E. (1980).   Sleep organization and motor development in prematures. In E.J. Sell (Ed.), *Follow-up of the high risk newborn: A practical approach* (pp. 187–193), Springfield, IL: Charles C. Thomas.

Barnard, K.E. (1978).   *Nursing Child Assessment Satellite Training Project Learning Resource Manual,* Unpublished program materials.

Barnard, K.E. & Bee, H.L. (1982).   *The assessment of parent-infant interaction by observation of feeding and teaching.* (Available from NCAST, CDMRC, WJ-10 University of Washington, Seattle, *WA* 98195).

Barnard, K.E, Bee, H., Booth, C., Mitchell, S., Sumner, G., & Magyary, D. (1982).   Grant Proposal: *Clinical Nursing Models for Infants and Their Families,* National Institute for Mental Health, Grant #1 R01 MH36894-01.

Barnard, K.E., Bee, H.L., & Hammond, M.A. (1984).   Developmental changes in maternal interactions with term and preterm infants, *Infant Behavior and Development,* **7,** 101–13.

Barnard, K.E., Booth C., Mitchell, S., & Telzrow, R. (1983).   Final Report: *Nowborn Nursing Models,* Grant #1 R01 NU-00719–03, Department of Health and Human Services, Division of Nursing, Health Resources Administration.

Barnard, K.E., & Eyres, S.J. (Eds.) (1979).   *Child health assessment, part 2: The first year of life.* U.S. Department of Health, Education and Welface, PHS, HRA, BHM, Division of Nursing, DHEW Publication No. (HRA) 79–25, Hyattsville, Maryland.

Beckwith, L., & Cohen, S.E. (1980).   Interactions of preterm infants with their caregivers and test performance at age 2. In T.M. Field, S. Goldberg, D. Stern, & M. Sostek (Eds.), *High-risk infants and children: Adult and peer interactions,* New York: Academic Press.

Beckwith, L., & Cohen, S.E. (1983, April).   *Continuity of caregiving with preterm infants.* Report presented at the Society for Research in Child Development, Detroit, Michigan.

Bee, H.L., Barnard, K.E., Eyres, S.J., Gray, C.A., Hammond, M.A., Spietz, A.L. Snyder, C., & Clark, B. (1982).   Prediction of IQ and language skill from perinatal status, child performance, family characteristics, and mother-infant interaction, *Child Development*, **53**, 1134–56.

Bradley, R.H., & Caldwell, B.M. (1976). The relation of infants' home environments to mental test performance at 54 months: A follow-up study, *Child Development*, **47**, 1172–74.

Brandt, P., & Weinert, C.A. (1982). Personal resources questionnaire—A social support measure, *Nursing Research*, **30**, 227–80.

Bromwich, R., & Parmelee, A. (1979). An intervention program for preterm infants. In T. Field, A. Sostek, & H.H. Shuman (Eds.), *Infants born at risk*, New York: Spectrum.

Brown, J.V., & Bakeman, R. (1979). Relationships of human mothers with their infants during the first year of life: Effect of prematurity. In R.W. Bell & W.P. Smotherman (Eds.), *Maternal influences and early behaviour*, New York: Spectrum.

Caldwell, B.M., & Bradley, R.H. (1978). *Manual for the Home Observation for Measurement of the Environment*, Little Rock, Arkansas: University of Arkansas.

Divitto, V., & Goldberg, S. (1979). The development of early parent-infant interaction as a function of newborn medical status. In T. Field, A. Sostek S. Goldberg, & H.H. Shuman (Eds.), *Infants born at risk*, New York: Spectrum.

Field, T.M. (1977). Effects of early separation, interactive deficits, and experimental manipulations on infant-mother face-to-face interaction, *Child Development*, **48**, 763–71.

Field, T.M. (1980). Interactions of preterm and term infants with their lower- and middle-class teenage and adult mothers. In T.M. Field, S. Goldberg, D. Stern, & M. Sostek (Eds.), *High-risk infants and children: Adult and peer interactions*, New York: Academic Press.

Field, T.M. Widmayer, S.M., Stringer, S., & Ignatoff, E. (1980). Teenage, lower-class mothers and their preterm infants: An intervention and developmental follow-up, *Child Development*, **51**, 426–436.

Frankenburg, W.K., van Doorninck, W.J., Liddell, T.N. & Dick, N.P. (1976). The Denver Prescreening Developmental Questionnaire (PDQ), *Pediatrics*, **57**, 744–53.

Fuhrmann, P.J. (1984). *The effect of preterm infants state regulation on parent-child interaction*, Unpublished master's thesis, University of Washington.

Gairdner, D., & Pearson, J. (1971). A growth chart for premature and other infants, *Archives of Disease in Childhood*, **46**, 783–787.

Goldberg, S., Brachfeld, S., & Divitoo, B. (1980). Feeding, fussing, and play: Parent-infant interaction in the first year as function of pre-maturity and perinatal medical problems. In T.M. Field, S. Goldberg, D. Stern & M. Sostek (Eds.), *High-risk infants and children: Adult and peer interaction*, NY: Academic Press.

Hollingshead, A.B. (1975). *Four-factor index of social status*. Unpublished manual, Yale University.

Kang, R., & Barnard, K. (1979). Using the neonatal behavioral assessment scale to evaluate premature infants. In *Birth Defects: Original Article Series*, Vol. XV, No. 7, pp. 119–144. The National Foundation, Founda March of Dimes, New York: Alan R. Liss, Inc.

76   K.E. BARNARD *et al.*

Lobo, M. (1982). *Mother's and father's perception of family resources and their adaptation to parenthood.* Unpublished doctoral dissertation, University of Washington.

Lobo, M.L., Barnard, K.E., & Cooms, J. (1982). *Failure to thrive: A parent-child interaction perspective, a systems approach.* Unpublished manuscript, University of Washington.

Magyary, D. (1983). Cross-time and cross-situational comparisons of mother-preterm infant interactions, *Western Journal of Nursing Research*, **5**, 15–25.

Magyary, D. (1984). Early social interactions: Preterm infant-parent dyads, *Comprehensive Pediatrics Nursing*, **7**, 233–254.

Murtaugh, J. (1982). *A descriptive study of social support and depression in low income women.* Unpublished master's these, University of Washington.

Parmelee, A., & Littman, B. (1974). *Perinatal Factor Scores.* Unpublished manuscript, University of California at Los Angeles Medical School, Department of Pediatrics.

Pless, I.B., & Satterwhite, B. (1973). A measure of family functioning and its application, *Social Science & Medicine*, **7**, 613–21.

Roberts, C.S., & Feetham, S.L. (1982). Assessing family functioning across three areas of relationships, *Nursing Research*, **31**, 264–69.

Ross, G. (1984). Home intervention for premature infants of low income families, *American Journal of Orthopsychiatry*, **54**, 263–270.

Sameroff, A. (1981). Longitudinal studies of preterm infants. In S. Freidman & M. Sigman (Eds.), *Preterm birth and psychological development*, New York: Academic Press.

Telzrow, R.W., Kang, R., Mitchell, S.K., Ashworth, C.D., & Barnard, K.E. (1982). An assessment of the behavior of the premature infant of forty weeks conceptional age. In L.P. Lipsitt & T.M. Field (Eds.), *Perinatal risk and newborn behavior*, Norwood, New Jersey: Ablex.

Thomas, R., & Barnard, K.E. (1986). *Family measurement study, zero to three.* Washington, D.C.: National Center for Clinical Infant Programs.

Weiss, R. (1979). The fund of sociability, *Trans-Action*, July/August, 36–43.

The effects of early mother-child interaction and maternal language patterns on later development

NORMA M. RINGLER

Case Western Reserve University/University Hospitals

A summary of some research on the effects of early and extended contact of primiparous lower socio-economic black mothers with their infants during the first three hours and the following three days after birth is presented. Results of verbal interaction over time include the relationship of mother's speech to their one and two year olds, the relationship of speech to the two year old with the speech and language comprehension of the children when five, as well as the acquisition of meanings through social interaction at two and five. The questions addressed are: are altered hospital procedures which resulted in significantly more attentiveness of mothers with newborns reflected in mother's use of language? Does maternal talk to children have a lasting effect on language development? What are the implications of study results for nurseries, home, early childhood curriculum, hospitals and school behaviors?

INTRODUCTION

In 1970 a study to determine whether hospital practices for the mothers of full-term infants influenced later maternal behavior was begun at the department of pediatrics, School of Medicine, Case Western Reserve University (Klaus, Jerauld, Kreger, McAlpine, Steffa, & Kennell, 1972).

To test the hypothesis that there is a period shortly after birth that is uniquely important for the mother-to-infant attachment, 28 primiparous women were placed in two study groups shortly after delivery of normal fullterm infants. Fourteen mothers (control group) had the usual physical contact with their infants (a glimpse of the baby shortly after birth, brief contact and identification at six to twelve hours, and visits for 20 to 30 minutes every four hours for bottle feedings). Fourteen mothers (extended contact) had 16 hours of additional contact. Mothers' backgrounds and infants characteristics were similar in both groups. The extended contact mothers were given their nude babies with a heat panel overhead for one hour within the first three hours after birth plus five extra hours of contact each afternoon of the three days after delivery. Mothers in the control group also had heat panels placed over their beds. Nurses spent five hours per day with the control mothers to eliminate any influence from nurses who cared for the mother during the extended contact period.

The mean age, socio-economic and marital status, color, sex of the infant, and days of hospitalization are shown in Table I.

EFFECTS OF MATERNAL BEHAVIOR AT ONE MONTH

To determine if this short additional time with the infant early in life altered later behavior, mothers were asked to return to the hospital a month after delivery for three separate observations made between the 28th and 32nd postpartum days (Kennell, Jerauld, Wolfe, Chesler, Kreger, McAlpine, Steffa, & Klaus, 1974). A standardized interview, observation of maternal performance during a physical examination of the infant, and a filmed study of the mother feeding her infant were carried out. All mothers bottle fed their babies. Scoring of the interview and observation of maternal performance were rated from 0–3 where 3 represents optimal maternal interaction. The extended-contact group had scores of 2 and greater, whereas the control mothers were below 2 ($p < .05$ with the Mann Whitney U test).

Time-lapse films of the mothers feeding their infants were analyzed in detail for 25 specific activities from routine caregiving to measurements of maternal interest and affection. The range of score for the controls was 2–10 and for the extended contact group 7–12 ($p < .002$, by the Mann Whitney U test). When the interview questions and examination observation scores were combined, the extended-contact mothers showed significantly greater "en face" and fondling (11.6% compared to 1.6% in the control group).

TABLE I

Clinical and Socio-economic data for mothers and infants

Characteristics	Group	
	Extended Contact	Control
Number	14	14
Mother's age (mean)	18.2 years	18.6 years
Marital Status:		
Single	10	9
Married	4	5
Infant sex:		
Male	6	8
Female	8	6
Race		
Black	14	14
Birthweight (mean) g	3184 g	3074 g
Nurses' time (min/day)	13	14
Hospital stay (days)	3.8	3.7
Economic status:		
A. Housing: (7.0 = poorest housing)	6.7	6.5
B. Occupation: (7.0 = unskilled workers)	6.7	6.9
C. Education: (5.0 = reaching 10th to 11th grade in high school)	4.9	4.9

At one month, extended contact mothers picked up their babies more frequently in response to crying, had a greater tendency to stay home with their infants, were observed to be more comforting during stressful office visits, and showed more fondling and increased eye contact during filmed feedings. Studies by Rubenstein (1967) and Bell (1970) indicated that increased maternal attentiveness facilitated later exploratory behavior and the early development of cognitive behavior in infants. Perhaps, then, early and extended contact for the human mother can have a powerful effect on her interaction with her infant and consequently on her baby's later development.

Study results suggest there may be a special sensitive period for the human mother. The early presentation of a baby shortly after birth may be perceived by a mother as a special privilege or recognition that alters her behavior and this altered behavior can extend for at least one month after delivery (Klause, *et al.*, 1972; Kennell *et al.*, 1974).

EFFECTS OF EXTENDED NEONATAL CONTACT ON MOTHER-INFANT INTERACTION AT ONE YEAR

When the infants were one year old, the 28 mother-infant pairs returned to the hospital for a second time for 1½ hours of observation (Kennell *et al.*, 1974). A physical examination of the infant and an interview were conducted and again results showed distinct differences between the behavior of the mothers in the two groups. Of the 6 extended contact mothers who had returned to work or school, five were more preoccupied with their babies, while one of the seven control mothers who had returned to work or school showed preoccupation with her baby (p<.05). During the physical exam, extended-contact mothers spent more time at the examination table assisting the physician (p<.05). They soothed more in response to the child's crying (50% vs. 25%) (p<.05), and also kissed the child more (p<.05). The mean score for the Bayley mental index was 98 for infants for extended-contact mothers and 93 for control infants (p<.05).

A comparison was made of maternal talk to adult examiners and to the children at age one and age two (Ringler, 1973). Rate of speech was significantly slower to child compared to adults. Maternal utterance length and correct grammar increased with child age. Speech to the child was simpler with less variety of vocabulary and less complex structure. There were more imperatives, action words, affirmatives and questions addressed to the child. Children received more verbal repetitions than adults.

Speech to children was more concrete with more nominatives and place adverbs.

Results suggested that mother's speech to children was different from that to an adult interviewer, that nursery language changed as the child began to talk, and children's speech probably influenced the mother's speech.

Armed with these comparisons a study was done of the linguistic behaviors of each group when the children were one year old and again when two years old.

LINGUISTIC BEHAVIORS OF MOTHERS WITH ONE YEAR OLDS

When the children were one year olds, maternal linguistic behavior indicated that the patterns of speech used by the two groups to their year-old children differed in only one respect (Ringler, Kennell, Jarvella, Navojosky, & Klaus, 1975). The extended-contact group used fewer statements ($p<.05$). Since one year old children are quite immature linguistically, it was not surprising that mothers in each group spoke to their children infrequently and used shorter utterances and a smaller assortment of utterances.

LINGUISTIC BEHAVIORS OF MOTHERS WITH TWO YEAR OLDS

When the children were two year olds, five mother-infant pairs were randomly selected from each of the two original groups of 14 mother-child pairs. Of the 1½ hours of different observations, results of the 15 minute free play period (mother and child alone) for the six girls and four boys are reported. Utterance sequences were classified according to a number of standard linguistic criteria yielding measures of rate, length, and variety of utterances. (Ringler *et al.*, 1975).

Table II notes significant differences between the two groups.

Mothers in the extended-contact group used fewer content words (words giving basic information, as in a telegram), and more adjectives. They also used more than twice as many questions and expressed significantly fewer commands than the control group

TABLE II

Characteristics of Mother to Child Speech at One and Two Years

Measure	One Year		Two Years	
	Extended Contact	Control	Extended Contact	Control
Number of words per proposition	3.43	4.34	4.62*	3.66
Mean utterance length	2.5	2.7	3.9	3.1
Percentage of:				
adjectives/all words	0.20	0.10	16.00**	12.00
content words/all words	62.40	57.60*	48.00	62.00**
questions/sentences	10.40	25.20	41.00*	19.00
imperatives/sentences	68.00	49.00	43.00	74.00*
statements/sentences	15.00	26.00*	16.00	6.00

*$p<.05$
**$p<.02$

mothers. The speech of the extended-contact mothers consisted of more appropriate forms for imparting information, for eliciting a response from the child, and for elaborating on simple concepts, indicating a wider repertoire of utterances. They also initiated more teaching behavior and provided more productive feedback language by asking questions with more complex sentence structures.

Mothers in the control group used more content words, rather than descriptors, and more imperatives (indicating more controlling behavior).

Extended-contact mothers had a greater awareness of the growing needs of their children. They assessed and interpreted the widening external environment as their children became older. They said more to the children that was illustrative and complex (use of adjectives, adverbs, conjunctions, and prepositions). This increased sensitivity and increased attention may have significant bearing on children's future cognitive and linguistic development.

THE RELATIONSHIP OF MATERNAL SPEECH TO TWO YEAR OLDS WITH CHILD DEVELOPMENT AT FIVE YEARS

Two groups of five year olds (n = 18) and their mothers were randomly selected from the 28 mother-infant pairs of the original longitudinal study of the effects of early and extended-contact in the postpartum period on later maternal attachment and child development. Measures of number of words per proposition, part of speech, and type of sentence function were included in the analysis comparing how mothers' speech at two might affect child speech and language comprehension at five.

The children at five were assessed using four standard tests (Ringler, Trause, Klaus, Kennell, 1978). Table III shows that five year old vocabulary comprehension (p<.01) was significantly related to the number of words per proposition used by the mothers when their children were two.

Experimental mothers who earlier used more adjectives had children who later comprehended more complex syntactic structure (p<.01). Mothers who earlier used more elaborate and illustrative speech had children who later had greater expressive ability (p<.01). Mothers who asked more questions of their two

TABLE III

Relationship of Maternal Speech at Two Years with Child Language Ability at Five Years for the Early Contact Group

Maternal Speech 2 Years n = 9		Child Performance 5 Years n = 9
A. Number of words per proposition	1. 3 Critical Elements	r = .76; p<.008
	2. 4 Critical Elements	r = .89; p<.001
B. Number of adjectives	1. I.Q.	r = .75; p<.009
C. Fewer content words (Illustrative speech)	1. Expressive ability	r = .76; p<.01
	2. Receptive ability	
	3 Critical elements	r = .81; p<.004
	3. 2 Critical elements	r = .87; p<.001

year olds had 5 year old children with somewhat higher IQ's, comprehension, and expressive ability (p<.01).

When their children were two years of age, the extended contact mothers used more adjectives, questions, words per proposition, and fewer content words and imperatives than control mothers. Significantly, the five year old children of the early contact mothers comprehended more complex phrases with four critical elements (p<.005), indicating greater maturity in syntactic development than children of control mothers. Thus, results suggest that the early linguistic environment of the young child, which may be altered by hospital practices at birth, appears to affect the child's speech and language comprehension at five years of age.

RELATIONSHIP OF MEANINGS IN MOTHER AND CHILD LANGUAGE AT AGE 2

When the children were two years old, the free play situation was further analyzed to determine the relationship of meanings, expressed as verbal interaction in social context and acquisition of language (Ringler, 1975;1980). The speech patterns of each mother-child pair were examined in a free play situation according to Halliday's basic function of alternative meaning potentials design (Halliday, 1973; 1975). The relationship of each mother's semantic pattern (in initiated speech and in response) to the child's developing expressive and meaning systems was examined.

MATERNAL LANGUAGE MEANING CATEGORIES

Mothers who had early and extended contact with their new borns were less controlling with their two year olds than control group mothers (See Table IV). They used significantly less (½ as much) regulating language (p<.01). They responded 13 times more with friendly verbal interactions with their two year olds than did control mothers. They also asked over twice as many questions and were more informative. Thus the experimental group mothers were less controlling, friendlier in responses, asked more questions,

TABLE IV

Category Means for Selected Language Functions of Parents and Two Year Old Children

Selected Categories of Language Function	Means			
	Child		Mother	
	Experimental	Control	Experimental	Control
Regulatory (Specific Commands)			.224	.483**
Total Regulatory			.312	.654**
Interactional (Friendly responses)	.060	.018	.075	.006**
Personal (awareness of self; personal feelings)			0.0	.013
general interest (non-specific references)				
Heuristic (questions)	.140	.078	.319	.128
Informative (Information given in communication)	.305	.144*	.187	.111
Babbling (Unintelligible speech)	.155	.389		

NOTE: Variables not mutually exclusive.

*$p < .05$
**$p < .01$

and were more informative with their two year olds than control mothers.

CHILD LANGUAGE MEANING CATEGORIES

Table IV shows that experimental two year olds were three times as friendly in their responses, and gave twice as much information as control two year olds. They also babbled less. Experimental mothers' use of friendly *responses* correlated positively with the two year old friendly *responses*. Maternal *initiation* of friendliness, however, correlated with their child responding in an unfriendly way, perhaps with two year old defiance, not uncommon for the age. *Maternal information* correlated positively with child's *friendly response*. Maternal commands were associated with unfriendly child vocalization and babbling. Experimental mothers used far fewer commands than the control group mothers, and used a variety of other meaning interactions more. For example, there was a trend for them to give more information than control group mothers. It can be seen in Table IV that control children gave fewer friendly responses and fewer information responses, and showed a trend for more unintelligible speech acts with their mother compared to experimental children.

Thus, results suggest that early and extended contact and early interactions of mother-child pairs as far back as the immediate postpartum periods relates significantly with two year old children's development of language and use of meanings.

CATEGORIES OF MEANING FOR MOTHER-CHILD LANGUAGE AT 5 YEARS

When the children were 5 years old, 6 mother-child pairs were randomly selected from the original group of low-income mothers who had participated in the longitudinal study of the effects of postpartum contact. Earlier data as stated suggested that the richer the mother's speech to her two year old (as reflected in the number of adjectives she used) the higher was the child's IQ at five. The longer her length of utterance to her two year old, the better the 5 year old child understood complex phrases. In contrast, the simpler and more telegraphic her speech (that is, the more content words she used), the poorer the five year old's expressive ability and comprehension of complex phrases.

MATERNAL LANGUAGE MEANINGS AT AGE 5

Table V shows that mothers who had early and extended contact were one-half as controlling with their pre-schoolers as mothers of five year olds who had limited postpartum contact with their newborns ($p<.05$). Experimental mothers initiated significantly less friendly behavior ($p<.01$) to their five year olds and showed trends of sharing less information with them.

CHILD'S LANGUAGE MEANINGS AT 5

The experimental child at five responded with friendliness more than $2\frac{1}{2}$ times that of the control child ($p<.05$), had self-awarness and shared feelings 17 times more ($p<.01$), and had a total interaction score twice that of the control child ($p<.05$). (See Table V). The extended contact children at 5 years showed five times more imagination than the control child, and a total personal function score three times that of the control child's.

The five-year-old experimental child was outgoing, responsive, friendly, interacted well, was very self-aware, shared feelings openly, and tended to be imaginative, but not informative. The experimental mother was less controlling, less friendly, asked many more questions than the control mother.

In both groups, experimental and control, maternal friendly response meanings were met with friendly behavior by their children. In the control group however, maternal commands correlated with the child's more submissive behavior. Maternal use of commands correlated negatively with the control child's use of information and questions. The experimental mother used three times fewer prohibitions with her five year old than control mothers.

TABLE V

Category Means for Selected Language Functions of Parents and Five Year Old Children

Selected Categories of Language Function	Means			
	Child		Mother	
	Experimental	Control	Experimental	Control
Regulatory (General Commands)	.06	.05	.060	.155**
(Specific Commands)	.03	.05	.139	.143
Total Regulatory	.095	.107	.199	.298
Interactional (Initiating friendly speech)	.070	.050	0.0	.056***
(Responding with friendliness)	.085	.032*	.117	.110
Total Interactional	.158	.083	.123	.166
Personal (awareness of self personal feelings) Interest-general (not specific)	.052	.003**	.035	.008
Total Interest	.088	.034	.053	.064
Total Personal references	.092	.037	.065	.023
Heuristic (questions)	.265	.201	.405	.217
Informative (Information given in communication)	.279	.512	.196	.295
Imaginative (Creative:—"let's pretend")	.107	.030	.011	0.0
Babbling (Unintelligible speech)	0.0	.029	0.0	0.0

*p<.05
**p<.01
***p<.009
NOTE: Variables not mutually exclusive.

Early and extended maternal information modes correlated with questions from the child; in turn, maternal use of questions correlated with her child's use of information. It seemed as if the experimental mothers' use of meaningful linguistic functions relating to cognition correlated with their five year olds' use of information and questions in a most appropriate way. In the control group the maternal use of information had low correlation with child questions.

In summary, among this small group of mother-child pairs, data at 5 years suggest that mothers in the mother-child dyads with extra and extended contact were less controlling. They no longer responded in a friendly way as they had when their children were 2, and they had less interaction and used less information in their communication.

The experimental children at 5 were more than twice as responsive and friendly as the control children, expressed feelings and self-awareness 13 times more, tended to use less information in communication, continued, as they had been at 2, to be friendly in their responses as compared to the control children. They also expressed emotions more and had more self-awareness. It might be that, despite the small sample, early shared meanings between parents and children affect later personality development.

EFFECTS OF POSTPARTUM CONTACT AND EARLY MATERNAL LANGUAGE AT AGE 8

Currently we are studying differences in classroom behavior and adjustment between two groups of children (8 experimental, 9 controls) randomly selected from the original 28 dyads study. The Devereaux Elementary Behavior Scale, which identifies overt potential problem behavior, has been used by their second grade classroom teachers as children approach their 8th birthday, to evaluate emotional and interpersonal behavior.

Children who had 16 additional hours of early and extended contact with their mothers at birth and who experienced richer and more complex language, less controlling maternal behavior, and more

D

freedom to express themselves, at eight shared more feelings and personal incidents than control children. They had less anxiety about achievement, were more independent in performing their school work, coped with authority better, and obeyed directions better. They also checked on the quality of their own work and followed it to completion. They had closer and more positive personal involvement with their teachers and peers.

Results of these studies continue to indicate that early and extended contact at birth, and the language patterns it fosters, seems to affect the child's ego development, learning, and behavior well into the future.

We must consider, however, that what we may be seeing is a consistency in patterns that hospitals can allow to get started at an early and sensitive period. It may be that these positive patterns of attentiveness and responsiveness become habitual modes of mother-child interaction building ego resilience and strength, autonomy, and a well attached child. With positive support of the continuance of positive patterns, (rather than a change in them—eg. noxious, less friendly interaction) we may be seeing the effects of stability in families, a consistency of patterns set in motion at a critical period when mothers first fall in love with their newborns.

References

Bell, S. (1970).   The development of concept of object as related to infant-mother attachment. *Child Development*, **41**, 291–311.
Halliday, M.A.K. (1973).   *Explorations in the functions of language*, London: Edward Arnold.
Halliday, M.A.K. (1975).   Learning how to mean. In E.H. Lenneberg (ed.), *Foundations of Language Development* (pp. 239–65). New York: Academic Press.
Halliday, M.A.K. (1975).   *Learning How to Mean: Explorations in the Development in Language*, London: Edward Arnold.
Kennell, J.H., Jerauld, R., Wolfe, H., Chester, D., Kreger, N.C., McAlpine, W., Steffa, M., and Klaus M.H. (1972).   Maternal behavior one year after early and extended post-partum contact, *Developmental Medicine and Clinical Child*, **16**, 172–79.
Klaus, H.M., Jerauld, R., Kreger, M.C., McAlpine, W., Steffa, M., Kennell, J.H. (1972).   Maternal attachment: importance of the first post-partum days, *New England Journal of Medicine*, **286**, 486–93.

Ringler, N. (1973).   Mothers' language to their young children and to adults over time. Unpublished doctoral dissertation, Case Western Reserve University, Cleveland.

Ringler, N.M., Kennell, J.H., Jarvella, R., Navojosky, B., Klaus, M.H. (1975).   Mother-to-child speech at two years: effects of early postnatal contact, *Journal of Pediatrics*, **86,** 141–44.

Ringler, N.M., Kennell, J.H., Jarvella, R., Navojosky, B., Klaus, M.H. (1975).   Mother-to-child speech at two years: effects of early postnatal contact, *Child Language*, **27,** 51–56.

Ringler, N.M., Trause, M.A., Klaus, M. Kennell, J. (1978).   The effects of extra post-partum contact and maternal speech patterns on children's IQ's and speech and language comprehension at five, *Child Development*, **49,** 862–65.

Ringler, N. (1978).   Mother-child reciprocity: its effect on affective behavior, meaning, and the development of language. In F. Peng, P. French (Eds.), *The Development of Meaning*, (pp 39–46) Hiroshima, Japan: Bunka Hyoron Publishing Co.

Ringler, N. (1980).   The effects of post-partum mother-infant reciprocal transactions on the development of meanings and language. Proceedings of the First International Congress for the Study of Child Language. Ingram, Peng, Dale. University Press of America.

Ringler, N., Melillo K., Stienke, L. (1982).   Development of meanings through parent child interaction. In R. St. Clair, W. Von-Raffler-Engel (Eds). *Language and Cognitive Styles* (pp. 283–291), Rotterdam: Swets & Zeitlinger-Leisse.

Ringer, N. (1983, March).   The effects of post-partum mother-infant reciprocal transactions on the development of language in 5 year olds. *World Congress on Infant Psychiatry Symposium*, Cannes, France.

Ringler, N., & Finlon, M.A. (1986, August).   Effects of postpartum contact and early maternal language patterns on development and learning at age eight. *Third World Congress on Infant Psychiatry and Allied Disciplines: Symposium*, Stockholm, Sweden.

Early environment and cognitive competence: The Little Rock study

ROBERT H. BRADLEY and BETTYE M. CALDWELL

Center for Child Development and Education University of Arkansas at Little Rock

Data from the Longitudinal Observation and Intervention Study (LOIS) were used to examine the relationship between early HOME scores (which measure parental responsivity, acceptance, involvement, provision of toys, variety of stimulation, and organization) in relation to cognitive scores of children at 1, 3, 4½, and 11 years of age. Partial correlations were run methodically to tease out the potential contributions of earlier and later HOME scores to the children's intellective and language functioning. The latter was assessed with the Illinois Test of Psycholinguistic Abilities. No difference in mean level of home stimulation for males or females was found, but there were differences in HOME scores as a function of race, SES, and family configuration. There is substantial relationship between HOME measures in first year of life and children's IQ scores at 3 and 4½ years. The correlations were stronger for white than for blacks. School performance at age 11 was linked to contemporaneous HOME scores, and thus to children's accumulating experiences more than to their early home experiences or their developmental status *per se.*

The decade of the 1960's was a watershed period in child development research. Few times in recent history have witnessed such a reshaping of our thinking about human development. The seminal volumes of Hunt (1961) and Bloom (1964) made clear the

---

Partial funding for the research reported herein was received from the Office of Child Development, the Office of Special Education Research, and the National Institute of Mental Health.

Thanks are offered to the families who have welcomed us into their homes for the purposes of collecting research data for this study. Thanks are offered, too, to those dedicated research assistants who have gone on thousands of home visits over the past 15 years. Their efforts have made this project not only possible but rich: Tricia Cromwell, Val Smith, Joan Rorex, Julie Honey, Beverly Hines, Ann Campbell, Pat Walter, Nina Lattimer, Shelvie Hawke, Pam Harris, Holly Hamrick, Ann Morgan, Joann Nelson, Loree Leslie, Judy Brisby, Jane Fitzgerald.

93

importance of the early environment for childhood development. The genetic epistemology of Piaget and Erikson's theory of psychosocial development molded new understandings of cognitive and social development. Theories of attachment caused a revolution in the thinking about early emotional development. Strict behavioral theories of learning gave way to social learning theories which recognized the place of intentionality and expectations in human behavior. Bell's (1968) work on the bidirectionality of influence between infant and caregiver foreshadowed currently esteemed transactional ecological and general systems models of human development. During this time major applications of child development theory were attempted, such as Head Start and a number of model early intervention projects (Caldwell and Freyer, 1983).

Out of the cataclysm of activity and research of the 60's two very critical ideas emerged. First, infants are competent, viable organisms who undergo qualitative changes in all spheres of development in the early months and years of life. Second, individual patterns of development for children result from a series of specific transactions between infant and environment, each shaping the other as the child displays increasingly complex and differentiated sets of capabilities and behaviors.

It was against this backdrop of child development research that the Longitudinal Observation and Intervention Study (Caldwell, Elardo, and Elardo, 1972) was set. The study, referred to as LOIS, commmenced in Little Rock, Arkansas in 1969. It was designed to explore the very important scientific question of when the decline in rate of development so often observed in children from disadvantaged backgrounds begins. A second purpose of the study was to explore the relation of the early home environment to development during infancy. Initial findings from the study (Elardo, Bradley & Caldwell, 1975; Bradley & Caldwell, 1976) prompted its continuation: to examine the relation of environment and development through later periods of childhood. It is the intent of this report to describe findings from the study from infancy to age ten.

METHOD

Sample

Recruitment of participants for LOIS began in November, 1970. Well-baby clinics, birth records from hospitals, and personal contacts in the community all served as sources of infants. Children were drawn from both middle class and lower class backgrounds. However, a disproportionate number were from poor families since that was the focus of the study. A total of 174 participants were recruited. General demographic characteristics for the sample are presented in Table I.

Not all of the participants were included in analyses of the relationship between home environment and children's develop-

TABLE I
Characteristics of the Little Rock Sample
(N = 174)

Family Data[1]		
Educational Status: (mean no. years)	Father = 12.9	Mother = 12.2
Employment Status:	Welfare = 59	Non-welfare = 115
	Wide range of employment but a high percentage fell into categories like semiskilled laborers or clerical	
Paternal Status:	Father present = 112	Father absent = 52
Child Data[2]		
Age Status:	4–12 months = 67	13–24 months = 59 25–36 months = 48
Race & Sex Status:	Black Males = 57 White Males = 31	Black Females = 58 White Females = 28
Birth Order Status:	First Born = 92 Fourth or later Born = 30	Second or Third Born = 52

[1] Complete data were not available on all families. Family data figures are estimates based on the available information.
[2] Complete birth order data were not available on all children. Birth order figures are estimates based on the available information.

ment. About half of the children were participants in one of the study's intensive intervention efforts. They were excluded for fear that results would be difficult to interpret. The analyses reported herein were done only on those children who did not receive intensive center based or home based intervention. Unfortunately, there has been substantial attrition over the ten years of the study, so that only 41 children participated at age ten.

INSTRUMENTS

Bayley Scales

All infants were administered the Bayley Scales of Infant Development up to age 24 months. All three of the Bayley Scales were used: the Mental Development Scale (MDI) the Motor Development Scale (PDI), and the Infant Behavior Record (IBR.)

Stanford-Binet

All children were administered the Stanford-Binet Intelligence Test at 36 and 54 months of age. Some were also administered the IQ test at 24 months.

Illinois Test of Psycholinguistic Abilities

All children were administered the Illinois Test of Psycholinguistic Abilities (ITPA) at 36 months.

SRA Achievement Battery

Around 40 children were administered the Science Research Associates Achievement Test battery in school at the age of 6 to 7 and again at the age of 10 to 11. The SRA tests were given to children as part of the school district's normal assessment routine for the year.

HOME Inventory

All families were administered the Home Observation for Measurement of the Environment (HOME) Inventory when the child was 6, 24, 36, and 54 months old. The Infant version of the HOME was given at the first three time points, the Pre-school version at the final two time points. The Infant HOME consists of 45 items clustered into six subscales: (1) parental responsivity; (2) acceptance of child; (3) organization of the environment; (4) play materials; (5) parental involvement with child; and (6) variety of stimulation. The Preschool HOME consists of 55 items clustered into eight subscales: (1) learning materials; (2) language stimulation; (3) physical environment; (4) pride, affection and warmth; (5) stimulation of academic behavior; (6) encouragement of social maturity; (7) variety of stimulation; and (8) physical punishment.

Classroom Behavior Inventory

41 children were rated using the Classroom Behavior Inventory at age 10 to 11. The CBI consists of 18 items clustered into three bipolar subscales: task orientation vs. distractability, consideration vs. hostility, and introversion vs. extraversion. Teachers rate the child on a 4-point scale for each item. They were also asked to appraise the child's overall adjustment using the same 4-point format.

Demographics

Basic demographic and family structure information was collected from all families. It was updated with each home visit.

RESULTS

Home Environment and Intelligence in the Preschool Years

A primary purpose of this report is to describe findings from the LOIS study as they pertain to the relationship between early environment and cognitive development. Included in Table II are correlations between HOME scores at 6, 12, and 24 months and the following measures of mental development: 12-month Bayley MDI, 36-month and 54-month Stanford Binet IQ.

Six-month HOME

Table II shows the Pearson product-moment and multiple correlation coefficients between HOME scores and Bayley Mental Development Index (MDI) scores at 12 months. The table also shows correlations between 6-month HOME scores and Stanford-Binet scores at 36 and 54 months. An examination of these coefficients indicates that variety in daily stimulation was correlated with the criterion r = .27. The multiple correlation between all six scores and the 12-month MDI scores was calculated at r = .30.

Correlations between 6-month HOME scores and 36-month Binet scores were generally higher than correlations between 6-month HOME scores and MDI performance at 12 months. This was particularly true of the relationship between 6-month HOME total score and 36-month Binet score (r = .50 vs. r = .16). It is also interesting to note that appropriate play materials (r = .41), maternal involvement (r = .33), organization of the environment (r = .40), and variety in daily stimulation (r = .31) were significantly related to 36-month Binet performance. The multiple correlation between 6-month HOME subscale scores and 36-month Binet IQ was computed at R = .54.

Correlations between 6-month HOME scores and 54-month IQ scores were very little different from correlations between 6-month HOME and 36-month IQ. The multiple R was still .50. For only two subscales was there a drop of as much as .10: acceptance of child (r = .10), organization of the environment (r = .31).

Twelve-month HOME

Pearson product-moment coefficients and multiple correlation coefficients between 12-month HOME scores and 12-month MDI scores and 36-month and 54-month Binet scores are shown in

TABLE II

Correlations between 6-, 12-, and 24-month HOME Scores and Mental Test Scores Gathered at 1,3, and 4½ Years

| HOME Subscales | Time of HOME Assessment | | | | | | | |
| | 6 Months | | | 12 Months | | | 24 Months | |
	1-yr. MDI[b]	3-yr. IQ	4½-yr.IQ	1-yr.MDI	3-yr.IQ	4½-yr.IQ	3-yr. IQ	4½-yr.IQ
Responsivity	.09	.25*	.27	.15	.39*	.34	.49*	.50*
Acceptance	.13	.24*	.01	.01	.24*	.21	.41*	.28*
Organization	.20	.40*	.31*	.20	.39*	.34*	.41*	.33*
Play Materials	.05	.41*	.44*	.28*	.56*	.52*	.64*	.56*
Involvement	.08	.33*	.28*	.28*	.47*	.36*	.55*	.55*
Variety	.27*	.31*	.30*	.05	.28*	.32*	.50*	.39*
Total Score	.16	.50*	.44*	.30*	.58*	.53*	.71*	.57*
Multiple Correlation[a]	.30	.54*	.50*	.40	.59*	.57*	.72*	.63*

*$p<.05$
[a] This represents the multiple correlation of all six HOME subscales.
[b] MDI—Mental Development Index from Bayley Scales.

Table II. The 12-month MDI scores were most related to appropriate play materials (r = .28) and maternal involvement (r = .28). A moderate relationship is also observed for organization of the environment (r = .20). A multiple correlation of R = .40 was found for six subscales and the 12-month MDI.

Correlations ranging from r = .24 to r = .56 were observed between 12-month HOME subscale scores and 36-month Binet scores, the highest being for appropriate play materials (r = .56) and for maternal involvement (r = .47). It was at 12-months that maternal responsivity also showed a strong relationship to mental test performance (r = .39). The correlation between 36-month Stanford-Binet scores and total 12-HOME score was found to be r = .58, while the multiple correlation between the six HOME subscales and Stanford-Binet scores was R = .59.

Correlations between 12-month HOME scores and 54-month Binet IQ scores were quite similar to those between 12-month HOME and 36-month Binet scores. The range was from r = .21 to r = .52 for the subscales, r = .53 for the total score, and a multiple correlation of R = .57. The only notable difference in the pattern of correlations for 4-1/2-year IQ scores as compared with 3-year IQ scores was for maternal involvement. For 36 months it was r = .47; for 54 months it was r = .36. This drop in r-value suggests that intellectual development requires continuous parental encouragement and involvement. Moreover, it suggests that the level of involvement may wax and wane in different families.

Twenty-four-month HOME

In Table II the correlations between 24-month HOME scores and 36-month Stanford-Binet scores are listed. Coefficients ranged from r = .41 for acceptance of child to r = .64 for appropriate play materials. The total HOME score at 24-months and the Binet score at 36 months share about 50% common variance (r = .71). The multiple correlation between the six HOME subscales and the 36-month Binet scores was computed at R = .72. A multiple R of 77 was computed when using HOME scores at 6, 12, and 24 months, and 36-month Binet scores.

All HOME subscale scores at 24 months were significantly correlated with 54-month Binet performance. These coefficients ranged from .38 for acceptance of child to .56 for appropriate play materials and .55 for maternal involvement. The multiple correlation was R = .63. In general these coefficients were slightly lower than those between 24-month HOME scores and 3-year IQ.

Delineating the Relationship of Early HOME and 3-year IQ

To examine the question of whether correlations between early HOME scores and later IQ represent the unique contribution of the early environment, or whether they result from the fact that early environment tends to be highly correlated with later environment, a series of partial correlations were performed. Specifically, 6-month HOME scores were correlated with 3-year IQ, controlling for 12-month HOME scores. Then 12-month HOMES scores were correlated with 3-year IQ, controlling for 6-month HOME scores. A similar set of partial correlations was done examining 12-month versus 24-month HOME scores. Separate analyses were done for males and females and for blacks and whites. Results of these analyses on combined race and sex groups can be found in Tables III–VI.

For females, no significant residual correlations between 6-month HOME scores and IQ were observed with 12-month HOME scores partialled out. By contrast, a significant partial correlation between 12-month HOME scores and IQ was observed when 24-month HOME was controlled. All 24-month HOME subscales revealed significant partial correlations with IQ when 12-month HOME scores were controlled.

For males, three of the six HOME subscales (organization of the environment, provision of appropriate play materials, and variety measured at 6 months showed significant partials with IQ when 12-month HOME scores were controlled. Almost the same picture emerged when partial correlations between 12-month HOME scores and IQ were calculated, regardless of whether 6-month or 24-month HOME scores were partialled out of the relationship, but maternal involvement was significant also.

TABLE III
Partial Correlations Between HOME Scores and 3-Year IQ

HOME Subscales	6-Month HOME and IQ Controlling for 12-Month HOME		12-Month HOME and IQ Controlling for 6-Month HOME	
	Male	Female	Male	Female
Responsivity	.19 (.37*)	.01 (.27)	.25 (.39*)	.49** (.54**)
Acceptance	.23 (.26)	.04 (.27)	.09 (.16)	.42** (.48**)
Organization	.34* (.50**)	.14 (.40*)	.25 (.46**)	.42** (.54**)
Play Materials	.46** (.62**)	.21 (.49**)	.64** (.74**)	.53** (.65**)
Involvement	.01 (.35*)	.12 (.47**)	.45** (.55**)	.49** (.64**)
Variety	.37* (.41*)	.21 (.30)	.14 (.23)	.37* (.43**)
Total HOME	.34* (.63**)	.05 (.55**)	.31* (.62**)	.51** (.70**)

NOTE: Simple correlations are displayed in parentheses.
* $p < .05$.
** $p < .01$.

TABLE IV
Partial Correlations Between HOME Scores and 3-Year IQ

HOME Subscales	12-Month HOME and IQ Controlling for 24-Month HOME		24-Month HOME and IQ Controlling for 12-Month HOME	
	Male	Female	Male	Female
Responsivity	.17 (.39*)	.30* (.54**)	.45** (.55**)	.35* (.56**)
Acceptance	.07 (.16)	.26 (.48**)	.27* (.30)	.45** (.58**)
Organization	.36** (.46**)	.25 (.54**)	.17 (.34*)	.37* (.59**)
Play Materials	.38** (.74**)	.26 (.65**)	.32* (.72**)	.53** (.74**)
Involvement	.29* (.55**)	.34* (.64**)	.45** (.62**)	.49** (.70**)
Variety	-.12 (.23)	.27 (.43**)	.45** (.49**)	.60** (.66**)
Total HOME	.17 (.62**)	-.06 (.70**)	.43** (.70**)	.65** (.84**)

NOTE: Simple correlations are displayed in parentheses.
*$p<.05$.
**$p<.01$.

TABLE V
Partial Correlations Between HOME Scores and 3-Year IQ

| HOME Subscales | 6-Month HOME and IQ Controlling for 12-Month HOME | | 12-Month HOME and IQ Controlling for 6-Month HOME | |
	Black	White	Black	White
Responsivity	−.01 (.04)	.26 (.39*)	.15 (.16)	.06 (.31)
Acceptance	−.10 (.05)	−.01 (.18)	.28* (.23)	.45** (.47**)
Organization	.48** (.52**)	.01 (.14)	.00 (.23)	.20 (.24)
Play Materials	.10 (.20)	.30* (.46**)	.41** (.45**)	.29* (.45**)
Involvement	−.07 (.09)	.25 (.46**)	.27 (.27)	.27 (.47**)
Variety	.14 (.08)	.48** (.40**)	−.28* (.26)	.10 (.12)
Total HOME	.09 (.25)	.39** (.58**)	.21 (.31)	.13 (.48**)

NOTE: Simple Correlations are displayed in parentheses.
* $p < .05$.
** $p < .01$.

TABLE VI

Partial Correlations Between HOME Scores and 3-Year IQ

HOME Subscales	12-Month HOME and IQ Controlling for 24-Month Home		24-Month HOME and IQ Controlling for 12-Month HOME	
	Black	White	Black	White
Responsivity	−.05 (.16)	.15 (.31)	.42** (.44**)	.28* (.38*)
Acceptance	.20 (.23)	.29* (.47**)	.15 (.19)	.22 (.44**)
Organization of-Environment	.15 (.23)	.05 (.24)	.16 (.23)	.34* (.41*)
Play Materials	.23 (.45**)	.20 (.45**)	.34* (.51**)	.25 (.47**)
Involvement	.14 (.27)	.30* (.47**)	.30* (.38*)	.34* (.49**)
Variety	−.38** (.26)	−.12 (.12)	.49** (.41*)	.37* (.37*)
Total HOME	−.13 (.31)	.09 (.48**)	.54** (.59**)	.36* (.57**)

NOTE: Simple Correlations are displayed in parentheses.

*$p < .05$.

**$p < .01$.

For blacks, a rather inconsistent pattern of partial correlations was obtained. At 6 months, only organization of the environment showed a significant partial correlation with 12-month HOME controlled. By comparison, correlations between three 12-month HOME subscale scores and IQ were noted with 6-month HOME scores partialled out (acceptance of child, provision of appropriate play materials, and variety of daily stimulation). Among the partial correlations between 12-month HOME subscales and IQ with 24-month HOME subscale scores controlled, only one subscale reached significance, variety of stimulation, and that was negative $(r = -.38)$. By contrast, four of the six subscales at 24 months showed significant partial correlations and the total HOME score had a very strong partial correlation $(r = .54)$.

For whites, the pattern of partial correlations is a bit more consistent. With 12-month HOME scores partialled out, the correlation between two subscales at 6 months and later IQ was significant (provision of appropriate play materials, variety of stimulation). A very strong partial correlation was observed between 12-month scores for acceptance of child and IQ with 6-month scores controlled $(r = .45)$. A significant partial was also obtained for provision of appropriate play materials. 12-month HOME scores from two subscales (acceptance of child and maternal involvement) showed significant partial correlations with 24-month scores controlled. All partials except two (acceptance of child and provision of appropriate play materials) were significant when 24-month HOME scores were correlated with 3-year IQ. Perhaps the most interesting finding was that 6-month total HOME score and 24-month total HOME score both had significant partials with IQ when 12-month HOME score was controlled; but the reverse was not true.

In an effort to explain more fully the results of the partial correlation analyses on combined groups, two additional types of statistical analyses were done. First, as with simple correlation analyses described earlier, partial correlations were performed separately on each of the four race-gender subgroups (WM, WF, BM, BF). Results of these analyses are contained in Tables VII and VIII. Second, autocorrelations between HOME subscale

TABLE VII
Partial Correlations between HOME Scores and 3-Year IQ

HOME Subscales	6-Month HOME and IQ Controlling for 12-Month HOME				12-Month HOME and IQ Controlling for 6-Month HOME			
	White Male	White Female	Black Male	Black Female	White Male	White Female	Black Male	Black Female
Responsivity	.18 (.34)	.34 (.45)	.09 (.12)	-.22 (-.10)	.15 (.33)	-.01 (.32)	.07 (.11)	.40 (.35)
Acceptance	.25 (.39)	-.18 (.02)	-.02 (-.02)	-.25 (.02)	.41 (.49)	.48 (.45)	-.05 (-.06)	.52 (.47)
Organization	-.12 (.03)	.27 (.28)	.66 (.61)	.20 (.33)	.37 (.36)	-.12 (.15)	-.32 (.07)	.40 (.47)
Play Materials	.53 (.59)	.06 (.34)	.28 (.39)	.17 (.26)	.32 (.44)	.38 (.49)	.54 (.59)	.32 (.37)
Involvement	.17 (.40)	.38 (.53)	-.06 (.05)	-.06 (.10)	.41 (.53)	.05 (.40)	.14 (.14)	.49 (.49)
Variety	.55 (.55)	.40 (.41)	.05 (.01)	.02 (.05)	.13 (.14)	.09 (.13)	-.50 (-.50)	.07 (.08)
Total Score	.41 (.61)	.37 (.55)	.29 (.33)	-.27 (.14)	.30 (.56)	.03 (.43)	-.03 (.18)	.59 (.55)

Coefficients in parentheses represent the simple correlation between HOME and IQ.
Coefficients > .40 are significant for simple correlations, > .41 for partial correlations.

TABLE VIII
Partial Correlations between HOME Scores and 3-Year IQ

HOME Subscales	12-Month HOME and IQ Controlling for 24-Month HOME				24-Month HOME and IQ Controlling for 12-Month HOME			
	White Male	White Female	Black Male	Black Female	White Male	White Female	Black Male	Black Female
Responsivity	.24 (.33)	.12 (.32)	.00 (.11)	.13 (.35)	.06 (.24)	.45 (.53)	.41 (.42)	.29 (.43)
Acceptance	.32 (.49)	.29 (.45)	−.05 (−.06)	.39 (.47)	.28 (.47)	.15 (.39)	.13 (.14)	.17 (.33)
Organization	.27 (.36)	−.21 (.15)	.04 (.07)	.28 (.47)	.15 (.29)	.53 (.52)	.08 (.10)	.24 (.45)
Play Materials	.33 (.44)	.03 (.49)	.28 (.59)	.23 (.47)	.17 (.35)	.41 (.61)	.27 (.59)	.35 (.45)
Involvement	.46 (.53)	.06 (.44)	−.08 (.14)	.43 (.49)	.37 (.46)	.39 (.53)	.33 (.35)	.44 (.51)
Variety	−.05 (.14)	−.16 (.13)	−.63 (−.50)	.09 (.08)	.21 (.24)	.57 (.56)	.48 (.22)	.69 (.69)
Total Score	.39 (.56)	−.33 (.43)	−.25 (.18)	.10 (.55)	.20 (.47)	.63 (.67)	.51 (.49)	.63 (.76)

Coefficients in parentheses represent the simple correlation between HOME and IQ.
Coefficients > .40 are significant for simple correlations, > .41 for partial correlations.

scores at 6, 12, and 24 months were calculated to determine the stability of each subscale.

An examination of the partial correlations for the four separate groups showed the following. Except for two subscales (acceptance of child and play materials), the significant partials for females between 12-month HOME scores and IQ controlling for 6-month HOME scores were primarily attributable to black females. As a matter of fact, the nonsignificant trends for white females on the remaining four subscales tended to show a greater residual correlation for 6-month than for 12-month HOME. Looking at the residuals for 24-month HOME scores, it appears that black and white females show nearly identical patterns. However, there is much greater difference between the 12-month and 24-month residuals for whites (see Table VI). For example, among white females the 12-month partials for organization of environment, variety of stimulation, and total score were −.21, −.16, and −.33, respectively. The corresponding partials at 24 months were .53, .57, and .63. As with the simple correlations, the partial correlations on combined groups were frequently higher—albeit not statistically.

In the case of males, one of the four significant partials for 6-month HOME was almost solely attributable to white males (see Table III), one to black males. Significant 12 months partials for maternal involvement and total score appear mostly due to white males. Moreover, in one instance where white males had a significant partial (acceptance of child), the combining of male subgroups reduced the correlation. The significant 24-month partial for maternal responsivity seems primarily due to black males, whereas the significant partial for acceptance of child seems primarily due to white males. Unlike the situation that obtained with females, the magnitude of correlations for the combined male group rarely exceeded the magnitude in at least one of the subgroups.

The sex differences observed are reminiscent of those recorded by Martin (1981), Baumrind (1979), and Bayley and Schaefer (1964). In all these studies, maternal warmth and responsivity appeared related to positive development outcomes in boys but not girls. According to Martin, a sense of control for boys may be a much more significant factor in the quality of their interactions, their willingness to explore the environment, and their achievement efforts. "It may well be that girls have an easier time in establishing mutually responsive, trusting and cooperative relationships with their mothers than do boys, so that control and lack of control are less salient interpersonal issues in the developing mother-daughter pair (Martin, 1981, p. 47)."

The partial correlation results for the four race-gender subgroups (see Tables VII and VIII) show that the significant 6-month partial for whites in play materials is most closely associated with white males. Similarly, the significant 12-month partials for maternal involvement in the case of white males was reduced to nonsignificance when both gender subgroups were combined. Among the most interesting results in the white subsample was the substantial difference in partials for the total HOME score, especially the 12-month partials, where 24-month HOME was controlled (.39 and −.33 for males and females respectively). Among the five significant 24-month partials recorded for whites, four were principally due to white females.

In the black subgroup, the significant 6-month partial for organization of the environment reflects black male performance. Among the significant 12-month partials, the one for acceptance of child reflects black females, the one for variety of stimulation reflects black males.

In an effort to delineate more fully the relative importance of consistency across time in the home environment versus the unique salience of the early period, the autocorrelations for each HOME subscale were examined. The stability of these six factors varied considerably across the four subgroups (BM, WM, BF, WF). For black males, there was little evidence for consistency for the HOME scores across the three time-points studied. Most coefficients were in the .2–.4 range. For black females there was little consistency from 6 to 12 months, slightly more from 12 to 24 months. The correlation between 12-month and 24-month total scores was .66. For white males, there was modest consistency across the three periods (a number of coefficients in the .3–.6

range. The greatest consistency observed was for white females. The correlation between 6- and 12- month total score was .76; between 12- and 24-month scores was .87. This finding suggests that white, mostly middle class, mothers find an acceptable, reasonably comfortable way of interacting with their daughters, one which is not much influenced by the daughter's behavior or other external factors.

Correlations with Language Performance

Closely related to studies of HOME and intelligence are studies of HOME and language development. Several investigators have examined this relationship. Our own study included 74 children and their families (48 black, 26 white). The sample was of heterogeneous SES, but a disproportionate number of children were from lower and lower middle SES families. For purposes of this investigation (Elardo, Bradley and Caldwell, 1977) HOME scores taken at 6 and 24 months were correlated with 37-month performance on the Illinois Test of Psycholinguistic Abilities (ITPA).

The Pearson Product-Moment and Multiple correlation coefficients for 6-month HOME scores and 37-month ITPA scores are displayed in Table IX. An examination of these coefficients reveals a substantial relationship between the two sets of variables. Variety in daily stimulation and appropriate play materials appear particularly salient for the early growth of language. The subscales maternal involvement and responsivity of mother also showed a strong relationship to several aspects of language, although their correlation with ITPA total score was not as significant. The types of stimulation assessed by HOME demonstrated a reasonably strong association with Auditory Reception, Auditory Association, Visual Association, Verbal Expression, and Grammatical Closure. The multiple correlation coefficients indicate that HOME subscale scores share between 18% and 21% common variance with these five psycholinguistic abilities. The multiple correlation for HOME subscales and the ITPA total scores was R = 41.

The Pearson product-moment and multiple correlation coef-

TABLE IX
Intercorrelations Among 6-month and 24-month HOME Scores and 37-month ITPA

Scores for the Total Sample[a]

ITPA Scales		Responsivity	Acceptance	Organization	Toys	Involvement	Variety	Total Score	Multiple R[b]
Auditory	6 mo.	.34**	.19	.32**	.37**	.32**	.28*	.46**	.47**
Reception	24 mo.	.42**	.27*	.38**	.62**	.53**	.44**	.60**	.65**
Visual	6 mo.	.29**	.14	.17	.27*	.21	.27*	.35**	.37
Reception	24 mo.	.36**	.28*	.25*	.45**	.39**	.31**	.47**	.48**
Visual	6 mo.	.13	.04	.20	.10	.14	.11	.17	.25
Memory	24 mo.	.17	.09	.09	.12	.04	.18	.14	.24
Auditory	6 mo.	.30**	.20	.29**	.37**	.28*	.25*	.43**	.43*
Association	24 mo.	.46**	.34**	.39**	.62**	.54**	.46**	.64**	.66**
Auditory	6 mo.	−.05	.02	.13	.09	.03	−.09	.04	.21
Memory	24 mo.	.28*	.05	−.01	.14	.14	.28*	.21	.37
Visual	6 mo.	.26*	.05	.24*	.37**	.31**	.35**	.41**	.46**
Association	24 mo.	.40**	.24*	.40**	.52**	.49**	.42**	.55**	.58**
Visual	6 mo.	.14	.09	.14	.12	.04	.01	.15	.19
Closure	24 mo.	.36**	.17	.10	.27*	.29**	.27*	.34**	.39
Verbal	6 mo.	.21	.18	.31**	.37**	.16	.22	.37**	.43*
Expression	24 mo.	.41**	.24*	.25*	.41**	.39**	.45**	.48**	.53*
Grammatical	6 mo.	.33**	.27*	.17	.29**	.25*	.41**	.41**	.44*
Closure	24 mo.	.42**	.45**	.35**	.57**	.51**	.62**	.62**	.63**
Manual	6 mo.	.22	−.11	.14	.21	.16	.22	.22	.37
Expression	24 mo.	.47**	.20	.22	.36**	.37**	.47*	.47**	.55**
Total ITPA	6 mo.	.28*	.13	.27*	.33**	.25*	.39**	.39**	.41*
Score	24 mo.	.52**	.30**	.32**	.55**	.51**	.61**	.61**	.65**

NOTE: [a]$n = 74$.
[b]This represents the multiple correlation of all six HOME subscales and ITPA scores.
*$p < .05$.
**$p < .01$.

ficients for 24-month HOME scores and 37-month ITPA scores are also displayed in Table IX. As expected, 24-month HOME scores show an even stronger association with 37-month ITPA scores than do 6-month HOME scores. In fact, all six HOME subscales and each of the ITPA subtests was significant. Responsivity of mother, appropriate play materials, maternal involvement, and variety in daily stimulation revealed the highest degree of relation to language growth. Variety in daily stimulation had the highest overall correlation to total language development ($r = .6$), whereas appropriate play materials showed highest relations with Auditory Reception, Auditory Association, Visual Association, and Grammatical Closure (coefficients ranged from .52 to .61).

Tables X and XI display correlations between HOME and ITPA scores for males and females, respectively. As expected, 24-month HOME scores are more strongly associated with 37-month ITPA scores than are 6-month scores. For males, maternal responsivity and play materials revealed the highest degree of relation to language capacity. Four aspects of language (auditory reception, auditory association, visual association, grammatical closure) produced the highest correlations with environmental quality. For females, all six HOME subscales were significantly correlated with language performance; the strongest relations observed were those for subscales play materials, involvement, and variety. Additionally, a greater number of significant correlations among HOME scores and psycholinguistic abilities appeared for females than for males. The sex differences obtained in this sample partially mirror those observed by Moore (1968). With due consideration for circularity of reasoning, language may be a more critical benchmark of adaptive functioning in girls, thus a more sensitive barometer of environmental quality. The relative ease with which many young girls enter into a mutually responsive, trusting relationship with parents (Martin, 1981) may have a "down side" for some girls. Some parents may become overly comfortable with the relationship and do little to encourage broader aspects of development. Rather than exposing young girls to a wide variety of people and events, they may, in fact, be somewhat more restrictive with exploratory and mastery

TABLE X

Intercorrelations Among 6-month and 24-month HOME Scores and 37-month ITPA

Scores for Males[a]

ITPA Scales		Responsivity	Acceptance	Organization	Toys	Involvement	Variety	Total Score	Multiple R[b]
				HOME Subscales					
Auditory	6 mo.	.38*	.25	.41**	.37*	.27	.42**	.51**	.61*
Reception	24 mo.	.45**	.04	.32*	.58**	.48**	.38*	.55**	.63**
Visual	6 mo.	.24	.19	.14	.17	−.01	.36*	.26	.48
Reception	24 mo.	.31	.11	.14	36*	.25	.23	.35*	.40
Visual	6 mo.	−.09	−.25	.27	.00	.11	.17	.03	.43
Memory	24 mo.	.00	.02	.05	−.07	−.16	.06	−.13	.28
Auditory	6 mo.	.39*	.22	.34*	.35*	.19	.37*	.46**	.56*
Association	24 mo.	.52**	.17	.29	.60**	.46**	.45**	.59**	.66**
Auditory	6 mo.	.00	.08	.25	.08	−.13	−.07	.05	.35
Memory	24 mo.	.38*	.18	−.10	.14	.03	.13	.20	.49
Visual	6 mo.	.38*	.15	.21	.39*	.25	.41**	.46**	.55
Association	24 mo.	.49**	.07	.31	50**	.43**	.39*	.52**	.59*
Visual	6 mo.	.07	.11	.17	.23	.03	.14	.19	.30
Closure	24 mo.	.47**	.26	.01	.24	.30	.14	.36*	.50
Verbal	6 mo.	.27	.11	.34*	.46**	.02	.15	.37*	.58*
Expression	24 mo.	.51**	.09	.13	.30	.25	.26	.38*	.54
Grammatical	6 mo.	.30	.19	.08	.12	.00	.39*	.25	.53
Closure	24 mo.	.44**	.28	.20	.49**	.41**	.31	.51**	.54
Manual	6 mo.	.18	−.23	.18	.15	.03	.21	.14	.48
Expression	24 mo.	.40**	.15	.22	.39*	.33*	.33*	.43**	.45
Total ITPA	6 mo.	.31	.13	.32*	.33*	.11	.35*	.39*	.52
Score	24 mo.	57**	.19	.23	.50**	.41**	.36*	.55**	.62**

NOTE: [a]$n = 38$.

[b]This represents the multiple correlation of all six HOME subscales and ITPA scores.

* $p < .05$

** $p < .01$

TABLE XI

Intercorrelations Among 6-month and 24-month HOME Scores and 37-month ITPA

Scores for Females

ITPA Scales		Responsivity	Acceptance	Organization	Toys	Involvement	Variety	Total Score	Multiple R[b]
Auditory	6 mo.	.32	.15	.20	.38*	.36*	.15	.41**	.41
Reception	24 mo.	.38*	.43**	.45**	.65**	.57**	.50**	.65**	.70**
Visual	6 mo.	.34*	.11	.19	.39*	.46**	.15	.43**	.48
Reception	24 mo.	.41**	.43**	.39*	.55**	.55**	.39*	.60**	.60*
Visual	6 mo.	.28	.22	.08	.18	.16	.05	.26	.31
Memory	24 mo.	.30	.13	.08	.27	.18	.09	.25	.36
Auditory	6 mo.	.22	.18	.23	.38*	.39*	.10	.39*	.42
Association	24 mo.	.40*	.50**	.52**	.65**	.61**	.48**	.69**	.69**
Auditory	6 mo.	−.10	−.03	−.02	.10	.19	−.10	.01	.31
Memory	24 mo.	.18	−.05	.07	.13	.22	.42*	.20	.50
Visual	6 mo.	.17	−.01	.24	.36*	.37*	.31	.36*	.47
Association	24 mo.	.31	.35*	.49**	.52**	.52**	.45**	.57**	.60*
Visual	6 mo.	.18	.07	.06	.01	.04	−.12	.10	.28
Closure	24 mo.	.25	.10	.15	.27	.26	.38*	.31	.44
Verbal	6 mo.	.16	.24	.24	.27	.32	.32	.37*	.50
Expression	24 mo.	.29	.37*	.38*	.52**	.52**	.65**	.58**	.69**
Grammatical	6 mo.	.35*	.32	.22	.43**	.45**	.22	.51**	.52
Closure	24 mo.	.39*	.56**	.49**	.64**	.58**	.50**	.69**	.70**
Manual	6 mo.	.24	−.03	.05	.26	.31	.11	.28	.40
Expression	24 mo.	.54**	.24	.19	.30	.40*	.60**	.50**	.74**
Total ITPA	6 mo.	.26	.12	.18	.33*	.38*	.17	.38*	.40
Score	24 mo.	.46**	.38*	.42**	.59**	.59**	.59**	.66**	.71**

HOME Subscales (spans the column header group)

NOTE: [a]$n = 36$.
[b]This represents the multiple correlation of all six HOME subscales and ITPA scores.
*$p<.05$.
**$p<.01$.

behavior—or at least less facilitating. A narrower range of behavioral competencies may be considered important for girls. For example, is there likely to be a sex difference in terms of how much the following areas of competence are valued for girls and boys? Psychomotor skills? Taking initiative in social encounters? Solving problems independently? Having knowledge of out-of-home events, situations, facilities?

In Tables XII and XIII the correlations between HOME and ITPA scores are displayed for blacks and whites, respectively. Substantial correlations between 24-month HOME scores and 37-month ITPA scores were observed for both races. It is only in the white sample, however, that significant correlations were obtained for 6-month HOME scores. Among blacks, responsivity, play materials, and variety appeared most strongly related to language competence; while among whites, responsivity, involvement and variety appeared most strongly related. Among whites, environmental quality, as measured by the HOME Inventory, was significantly related to 9 of the 10 psycholinguistic abilities tested, this figure being 5 out of 10 for blacks. The multiple correlation coefficient between the six HOME subscales at 24 months and the ITPA total score was somewhat higher for whites $(R = .74)$ than for blacks $(R = .57)$.

HOME ENVIRONMENT AND ACADEMIC ACHIEVEMENT

School Performance at Age Seven

Bivariate and partial correlational analyses were performed to determine the relation between early environmental scores and achievement test performance at the end of first grade. As Table XIV reveals, there were several significant correlations between 12-month HOME scores and later achievement. The most notable finding involved the subscale provision of appropriate play materials. Correlations between play materials and achievement ranged from .58 for reading to .44 for math. Four of the HOME subscales showed significant correlations with at least one achievement area. None were noted for maternal responsivity and

TABLE XII

Intercorrelations Among 6-month and 24-month HOME Scores and 37-month ITPA

Scores for Blacks[a]

ITPA Scales		Responsivity	Acceptance	Organization	Toys	Involvement	Variety	Total Score	Multiple R[b]
				HOME Subscales					
Auditory Reception	6 mo.	.14	.08	.23	.14	.21	.09	.22	.30
	24 mo.	.34*	.10	.17	.48**	.41**	.37**	.47**	.55**
Visual Reception	6 mo.	.11	.03	.02	.07	.07	.23	.13	.24
	24 mo.	.21	.16	.05	.31*	.15	.22	.28	.39
Visual Memory	6 mo.	.10	−.07	.22	.08	−.01	.28	.13	.42
	24 mo.	.09	−.04	−.01	−.00	−.07	.02	.00	.20
Auditory Association	6 mo.	.07	.11	.19	.13	−.12	.10	.17	.23
	24 mo.	.35*	.25	.23	.55**	.40**	.43**	.54**	.61**
Auditory Memory	6 mo.	−.25	.01	.18	.01	−.04	−.16	−.09	.37
	24 mo.	.26	−.02	−.07	.13	.02	.24	.15	.41
Visual Association	6 mo.	.20	.02	.07	.21	.13	.23	.23	.33
	24 mo.	.24	.14	.29*	.40**	.35*	.29*	.41**	.44
Visual Closure	6 mo.	.03	.06	.13	.09	.06	−.04	.08	.15
	24 mo.	.23*	−.00	−.07	.14	.13	.23	.21	.41
Verbal Expression	6 mo.	.01	.14	.18	.25	−.04	−.05	.13	.36
	24 mo.	.28	.06	−.02	.19	.18	.31*	.25	.39
Grammatical Closure	6 mo.	.12	.13	−.04	−.02	.06	.25	.11	.31
	24 mo.	.31*	.24	.12	.40**	.26	.31*	.41**	.48
Manual Expression	6 mo.	.07	−.27	.08	.02	.04	.15	.02	.37
	24 mo.	.40**	.13	.10	.28	.23	.40**	.38**	.51*
Total ITPA Score	6 mo.	.06	.02	.18	.13	.09	.14	.14	.22
	24 mo.	.44**	.14	.10	.41**	.30*	.40**	.45**	.57**

NOTE: [a]$n = 48$.
[b]This represents the multiple correlation of all six HOME subscales and ITPA scores.
*$p < .05$.
**$p < .01$.

TABLE XIII

Intercorrelations Among 6-month and 24-month HOME Scores and 37-month ITPA

Scores for Whites[a]

ITPA Scales		Responsivity	Acceptance	Organization	Toys	Involvement	Variety	Total Score	Multiple R[b]
Auditory Reception	6 mo.	.54**	−.03	−.03	.44*	.24	.37	.49**	.64
	24 mo.	.28	.06	.38	.63**	.50**	.41	.50*	.73*
Visual Reception	6 mo.	.54**	.09	.18	.43*	.22	.18	.49**	.57
	24 mo.	.48**	.22	.46*	.50**	.67**	.29	.59**	.69
Visual Memory	6 mo.	.05	.02	−.19	−.10	.22	−.38	−.04	.54
	24 mo.	.11	.08	−.03	−.06	−.03	.01	.03	.25
Auditory Association	6 mo.	.46*	.00	.05	.44*	.25	.26	.45*	.52
	24 mo.	.51**	.15	.33	.61**	.56**	.41	.58**	.73*
Auditory Memory	6 mo.	.57**	.12	.14	.41	.23	.14	.49**	.58
	24 mo.	.53**	.42*	.43*	.56**	.61**	.48**	.68**	.70*
Visual Association	6 mo.	.18	−.30	.06	.36	.30	.40	.33	.55
	24 mo.	.48**	−.01	.32	.47*	.48**	.48*	.50**	.69*
Visual Closure	6 mo.	.26	−.02	−.15	−.01	−.13	−.06	.03	.44
	24 mo.	.27	.33	.25	.37	.44*	.21	.42*	.48
Verbal Expression	6 mo.	.36	−.08	.18	.32	.17	.46*	.50	.55
	24 mo.	.43*	.15	.35	.39	.43*	.52**	.51**	.58
Grammatical Closure	6 mo.	.52*	.18	−.02	.41	.22	.18	.48**	.54
	24 mo.	.39	.57**	.40	.65**	.67**	.42	.69**	.77**
Manual Expression	6 mo.	.51**	.07	.07	.55**	.28	.35	.55**	.62
	24 mo.	.59**	.21	.47*	.53**	.60**	.53**	.66**	.70*
Total ITPA Score	6 mo.	.48**	−.05	.03	.39	.23	.27	.44*	.54
	24 mo.	.55**	.22	.42*	.62**	.65**	.46*	.66**	.74*

Note: [a] $n = 26$.
[b] This represents the multiple correlation of all six HOME subscales and ITPA scores.
*$p < .05$.
**$p < .01$.

maternal involvement. Correlations between the HOME total score and later achievement were quite similar to those for provision of appropriate materials.

In general, the partial correlations between 12-month HOME scores and first-grade achievement with 12-month MDI scores controlled were at essentially the same level as the simple bivariate correlations. However, when the effects of 3-year IQ were partialed out, little significant residual relation remained between 12-month HOME scores and first-grade achievement test scores. As Table XIV shows, only three significant partials were observed. Similarly, when 24-and 36-month HOME scores were partialed out, little residual relation remained.

When 24-month HOME scores were correlated with first-grade achievement, many significant relations were observed. Four of the six HOME subscales were moderately correlated with achievement ($r = .4$ to $.5$). Only maternal responsivity showed negligible correlations, while organization of the environment showed only a slight relation ($r = .3$). The 24-month total HOME score was correlated around $r = .6$, with all three achievement scores (see Table XV).

Partialing out 12-month MDI from the 24-month HOME/achievement relation revealed little change in the level of the correlation from that shown in simple correlations (see Table XV). However, partialing out 3-year IQ resulted in little residual correlation. The subscale acceptance of child did show a significant partial for all three achievement scores, as did the total HOME score. In the case of the 24-month total HOME score, a significant residual correlation was observed when the 36-month total HOME score was partialed out.

School Performance at Age Eleven

The most recent follow-up of LOIS children occurred when they were age 11. SRA achievement test scores were obtained from 41 children. In addition, the Classroom Behavior Inventory ratings were done by the teacher, and the Elementary School version of the HOME was administered in the home.

TABLE XIV

Correlations between 12-month HOME scores and First-Grade Achievement controlling for 12-month MDI, 3-year IQ, 24-month HOME and 36-month HOME.

(N = 37)

HOME Subscales	Achievement Scores		
	Reading	Language Arts	Mathematics
Responsivity[a]	.30	.14	.01
MDI[b]	.25	.08	−.05
MDI + IQ[c]	.23	.01	−.14
Acceptance[a]	.19	.29	.31
MDI[b]	.20	.30	.33*
MDI + IQ[c]	.10	.24	.27
Organization[a]	.38*	.32*	.19
MDI[b]	.36*	.29	.17
MDI + IQ[c]	.14	.06	−.10
Toys[a]	.58**	.47**	.44**
MDI[b]	.56**	.44**	.42**
MDI + IQ[c]	.36*	.19	.17
Involvement[a]	.25	.20	.04
MDI[b]	.21	.16	.00
MDI + IQ[c]	.00	−.06	−.26
Variety[a]	.32*	.39*	.15
MDI[b]	.30	.37*	.12
MDI + IQ[c]	.32	.40*	.09
TOTAL[a]	.56**	.47**	.33*
MDI[b]	.54**	.44**	.30
MDI + IQ[c]	.34*	.20	.02
24 and 36 mo. HOME[d]	.17	.08	−.21

[a]Simple product-moment correlation between HOME score and Achievement score.
[b]Partial correlation between HOME and Achievement controlling for 12-month MDI.
[c]Partial correlation between HOME and Achievement controlling for MDI and 3-year IQ.
[d]Partial correlation between HOME and Achievement controlling for later HOME scores.
*$p<.05$.
**$p<.01$.

TABLE XV

Correlations between 24-month HOME scores and First-Grade Achievement Scores controlling for 12-month MDI, 3-year IQ and 36-month HOME.

(N = 37)

HOME Subscales	Achievement Scores		
	Reading	Language Arts	Mathematics
Responsivity[a]	.30	.16	.27
MDI[b]	.27	.12	.24
MDI + IQ[c]	−.10	−.31	−.11
Acceptance[a]	.41**	.43**	.46**
MDI[b]	.39*	.42*	.45**
MDI + IQ[c]	.33*	.37*	.41*
Organization[a]	.35*	.31	.26
MDI[b]	.33*	.29	.24
MDI + IQ[c]	.13	.07	.02
Toys[a]	.55**	.53**	.49**
MDI[b]	.56**	.54**	.50**
MDI + IQ[c]	.22	.19	.16
Involvement[a]	.39*	.47**	.49**
MDI[b]	.39*	.47**	.49**
MDI + IQ[c]	.03	.16	.23
Variety[a]	.52**	.47**	.39*
MDI[b]	.51**	.45**	.37*
MDI + IQ[c]	.31	.23	.13
TOTAL[a]	.65**	.59**	.61**
MDI[b]	.64**	.58**	.60**
MDI + IQ[c]	.35*	.24	.32*
36-month HOME[d]	.30	.38*	.43**

[a] Simple product-moment correlation between HOME score and Achievement score.

[b] Partial correlation between HOME and Achievement controlling for 12-month MDI.

[c] Partial correlation between HOME and Achievement controlling for MDI and 3-year IQ.

[d] Partial correlation between HOME and Achievement controlling for later HOME·scores.

*$p<.05$.

**$p<.01$.

E

As Table XVI shows, there is remarkable consistency in the pattern of correlations obtained between HOME scores and SRA scores as compared to the achievement test results obtained when the children were age 7. Correlations based on 35 cases showed marginally significant relations between HOME subscale scores obtained when children were 6 months old and SRA achievement scores. Provision of appropriate play materials and maternal responsivity revealed the strongest correlations ($r = .27$ to $.28$). Interestingly, four of the six HOME subscales showed low correlations with the teacher's ratings of the child's overall school adjustment ($r = .25$ to $.35$). The highest correlation was with maternal involvement. Correlations between 24-month HOME scores and school achievement were not much different. Provision of appropriate play materials and maternal involvement showed marginal relationships with SRA scores ($.29$ to $.30$). None of the correlations with school adjustment reached statistical significance.

Elementary HOME scores and SRA scores were available for 39 children. Significant correlations were observed for two HOME subscales (provision for active stimulation and family participation in developmentally stimulating experiences) and composite SRA score. Significant correlations were observed between six of the eight HOME subscales and teacher's ratings of overall school adjustment ($r = .28$ to $.44$).

As was done with the earlier achievement test and mental test scores, an attempt was made to determine whether the significant correlations obtained between HOME scores and cognitive scores were primarily a function of the fact that early HOME scores had unique predictive value for achievement at age 11. Partial correlations between 6-month HOME scores and SRA scores were not significant when 11-year HOME scores were controlled. Neither was the partial between 2-year HOME scores and SRA scores once 11-year HOME was controlled. The reverse tended not to be true. That is, the partial correlation between 11-year HOME scores and SRA achievement test scores were significant when 6-month HOME was controlled ($.35$) and marginal when 2-year HOME was controlled ($.29$). Thus, it appears that *children's school*

TABLE XVI
Correlations between HOME Scores and School Performance at Age 11

HOME Subscales		SRA Composite	School Adjustment
Infant HOME			
Maternal Responsivity	6 mo.	.27	.26
	24 mo.	.09	.12
Acceptance of Child	6 mo.	.21	.25
	24 mo.	.02	.12
Organization of Environment	6 mo.	.16	.13
	24 mo.	.18	.23
Play Materials	6 mo.	.28	.31
	24 mo.	.30	.22
Maternal Involvement	6 mo.	.23	.35
	24 mo.	.29	.03
Variety of Stimulation	6 mo.	.07	.32
	24 mo.	.08	.20
TOTAL Score	6 mo.	.13	.21
	24 mo.	.27	.12
Elementary HOME			
Parental Responsivity		.21	.44*
Encouragement of Maturity		.14	.28*
Emotional Climate		.23	.03
Materials and Experiences		.19	.31*
Active Stimulation		.45*	.36*
Family Participation		.34*	.45*
Paternal Involvement		.01	.10
Physical Environment		.18	.34*
TOTAL Score		.38	.45

*p < .05

performance is most directly related to contemporaneous factors in the home environment—albeit partial correlations for specific subscales were not investigated in this study. In this context, it is interesting to note that 2-year HOME scores and 11-year HOME scores had virtually the same level of correlation with 3-year IQ (.56 vs. .57); and that the correlation between 3-year IQ and 11 year

SRA was lower than the correlation between 11-year HOME and 11-year SRA (.29 vs .38). Indeed, it was essentially the same as the correlation between 2-year HOME and 11-year SRA (r = .27). The partial correlation between 3-year IQ and 11-year SRA was insignificant when 11-year was controlled.

Results based on the data from the children at age 10 to 11 suggest that children's experiences gradually shape their behavior and development. Neither early environment nor early developmental status appears to have a predominant influence throughout childhood—except perhaps when early environment is extremely understimulating or unsupportive or when there is organic damage. There were too few cases, particularly cases having extremely low scores, to investigate this issue thoroughly. Overall, the partial correlations suggest the importance of *continuity of developmental support and stimulation.* Even though contemporaneous environmental factors appear most strongly associated with 11-year developmental scores, the partial correlations for 11-year HOME and SRA were clearly reduced when earlier HOME scores were controlled.

SUMMARY

In general, the series of investigations using the HOME Inventory based on the sample obtained in Little Rock may be summarized as follows.

There is a little evidence that the home environments of males and females differ in terms of the mean level of stimulation available during infancy.

There appears to be a moderate level of stability in the quality of stimulation available in the home environments of most children throughout infancy.

In terms of mean performance, there appear to be differences in HOME scores as a function of race, SES, and family configuration. However, there is evidence that many of the differences reflect the natural confound that exists between many of these demographic variables (i.e., black children tend to live more often in large families where there is little money and only one poorly educated parent who has limited social and economic support). When each of these demographic factors was examined controlling for all others, the degree of crowding and birth order appeared to account for the greatest variance in HOME scores, with SES, race, and gender contributing less. Over half the variance in HOME remained unaccounted for even when all the factors were added together.

There is a substantial relation between the HOME measures of cognitive development throughout the preschool period. Correlations with Bayley scores in the first year of life tend to be slight. However, correlations with IQ scores at 3 years and 4-1/2 years are moderate to strong (.4 to .7). Correlations between HOME and intelligence test scores tend to increase, the closer the timing of the environmental and developmental measures. Correlations between 24-month HOME scores and later IQ were stronger than those between 12-month HOME and later IQ.

There is some evidence for race and gender differences in the pattern of our correlations between HOME and later intelligence test scores. Correlations tended to be a little stronger for whites than for blacks and a little stronger for males than for females. However, the differences were more pronounced for correlations between 6-month HOME scores and later IQ than for 24-month HOME and later IQ. Furthermore, the race and gender differences tended to be restricted more to certain subscales rather than to the total HOME score. Correlations between HOME and IQ tended to be more independent of social status for blacks than whites. As Golden and Birns (1968) observed, there is wide variability in parenting practices within social class for black families. An interesting hypothesis relative to this observation is: parenting practices and class status within a culture tend to converge over time. However, for families that change status, the convergence may require several generations. Moreover, the convergence in a culture is only likely to be partial, leaving substantial within class variation in parenting.

Correlations between HOME and language performances were

similar to those between HOME and IQ. There were, however, more sex differences in the pattern of correlations for language than for general IQ.

There is evidence that the correlation between early environment and later IQ may reflect the fact that the quality of the home environment tends to remain stable across time and the fact that the later home environment is highly correlated with IQ. On the other hand, there is some (albeit lesser) evidence that certain early home factors may have a more lasting impact, independent of the intervening environment.

School performance appears to be linked to the quality of stimulation found in both the early environment and the contemporaneous environment. The relative influence of the early environment appears to diminish over time, as children's experiences change and accumulate. School performance, both achievement test scores and classroom behavior, appear to reflect the child's accumulating experiences more than early experience per se or early developmental status. There is also some support for Bloom's (1964) position that development is affected by how consistent the environment is across time.

References

Baumrind, D. (1979).   Sex-related socialization effects. Paper presented at the biennial meeting of the Society for Research in Child Development, San Francisco.

Bayley, N. and Schaefer, E. (1964).   Correlations of maternal and child behaviors with the development of mental abilities: Data from the Berkeley Growth Study. *Monographs of the Society for Research in Child Development*, **29** (6, Serial No. 97).

Bell, R. (1969).   A reinterpretation of the direction of effects in studies of socialization. *Psychological Review*, **75**, 81–95.

Bloom, B. (1964).   *Stability and change in human characteristics*, New York: Wiley.

Bradley, R. and Caldwell, B. (1976).   The relationship of infants' home environment to mental test performance at fifty-four months: A follow-up study. *Child Development*, **47**, 1172–1174.

Bradley, R. and Caldwell, B. (1980).   Home environment, cognitive competence and IQ among males and females, *Child Development*, **51**, 1140–48.

Bradley, R. and Caldwell, B. (1982).   The consistency of the home environment and its relation to child development. *International Journal of Behavioral Development*, **5**, 445–65.

Bradley, R. and Caldwell, B. (1984).   The relation of infants' home environments to achievement test performance in first grade: A follow-up study, *Child Development*, **55**, 803–809.

Caldwell, B., Elardo, R. and Elardo, P. (1972).   The longitudinal observation and intervention study. Paper presented at the Southeastern Conference on Human Development, Williamsburg, Virginia.

Caldwell, B. and Freyer, M. Day care and early education (1982).   In B. Spodek (ed.), *Handbook of research in early childhood education*, New York: Free Press.

Elardo, R., Bradley, R. and Caldwell, B. (1975).   The relation of infants' home environments to mental test performance from 6 to 36 months: A longitudinal analysis, *Child Development*, **46**, 71–76.

Elardo, R., Bradley, R. and Caldwell, B. (1977).   A longitudinal study of the relation of infants' home environment to language development at age three, *Child Development*, **48**, 595–603.

Golden, M. and Birns, B. (1968).   Social class and cognitive development in infancy, *Merrill-Palmer Quaterly*, **11**, 139–160.

Hunt, J. (1961).   *Intelligence and experience*, New York: Ronald.

Martin, J. (1981).   A longitudinal study of the consequences of early mother-infant interaction: A microanalytic approach. *Monographs of the Society for Research in Child Development.* **46** (3, Serial No. 191).

Moore, T. (1968).   Language and intelligence: A longitudinal study of the first eight years, part II, Environmental correlates of mental growth *Human Development*, **11**, 1–24.

Early mother-son relations and son's cognitive and social functioning at age 9: A twin longitudinal study

HUGH LYTTON, DENISE WATTS and BRUCE E. DUNN

The University of Calgary
Calgary, Alberta, Canada

A longitudinal study of twin boys examined how well mothers' and sons' characteristics and mutual interactions, assessed when the sons were 2, predict the sons' cognitive and social characteristics at age 9. Ratings of social characteristics were obtained at both ages from interviews with mother and cognitive abilities were also assessed at both ages. Cognitive competence could be predicted very well from the child's 2-year characteristics, particularly vocabulary IQ, and from mother's education level, which is seen as an index of her genetic contribution and environmental stimulation. However, her 2-year socialization practices predicted cognitive competence poorly. Some 9-year social characteristics, on the other hand, were fairly well predicted by mother's 2-year attitudes and practices, whereas the child's own disposition and mother's education level had only a small effect on them.

The question of the effects of parental treatment and child-rearing practices on children's development holds a perennial fascination, since most parents *want* to know how to influence their children for the good. Many investigations into these effects have appeared in the literature and these have been reviewed, for instance, by Clarke-Stewart and Apfel (1978). Most of the research suffers from two limitations: firstly, it makes the implicit assumption that the influence is unidirectional—from parents to child—and fails to take into account the child's influence on his parents' practices and thereby on his own development; and secondly, it confounds genetic and environmental effects, by not allowing for the influence of parental IQ both on the nature of the interaction and on the child's development. These two possible paths of influence—the influence from the child's disposition and that from parental intelligence—are, of course related. The child's influence on his own cognitive development has rarely been studied in combination with parental effects, but there are studies that have made allowance for parental IQ in various ways, and these have been reviewed by Rutter (1985).

The parent-child interactions that the literature has shown to be beneficial to cognitive advancement in the child are characterized by: a good deal of active interaction with the child, i.e., engaging in both play and conversation with the child by sharing and expanding the child's activities, providing a variety of play materials, being responsive to the child's verbal and nonverbal signals, making demands and holding expectations of the child's achievements and encouraging his independence, i.e., generally attempting to promote his cognitive growth, and, in the context of these demands, exercising moderate to severe discipline. While there is also a relationship between maternal affection and IQ, this is probably mediated by other variables, such as verbal interactions, stimulation and responsiveness, which have a more direct impact on the child's cognitive development and all of which are interrelated with warmth and affection (Clarke-Stewart & Apfel, 1978; McCall, Appelbaum & Hogarty, 1973; Rutter, 1985). Authoritarian and intellectually constrictive discipline, however, particularly if it is a manifestation of hostility and rejection, has an adverse effect on the child's cognitive advancement.

Some years ago the senior author started observing the interactions of 2-year-old twin and singleton boys with their parents in a naturalistic home setting, with the object of tracing the influence of these parent-child interactions, as well as of genetic factors, on the development of important social characteristics, and on verbal competence. The results of this enquiry were published in book form (Lytton, 1980). More recently we followed up this sample of twin boys at the average age of 9 years both by observation and interviews at home and by tests at school. Part of this investigation addressed the following questions: 1) to what extent mothers' and fathers' attitudes and behaviors, as seen in the parent-child interactions at age 2, would predict the cognitive competence and the social functioning and adjustment of the twin boys at age 9, 2) to what extent the child's own early attributes and interactive behavior would predict these characteristics, and 3) whether social and cognitive characteristics were equally predictable.

Special features of this longitudinal research are: the 2-year data are based on naturalistic observations of parent-child interactions; fathers', as well as mothers' interactions were observed and analyzed; we can compare the manner in which parental characteristics are related longitudinally to the child's cognitive versus his social characteristics; and the sample consists of twins. With respect to this last point it should be said that though we found differences between twins and nontwins in level of verbal ability and attainments (the twins being slightly lower), a finding that is in line with that of other investigations (e.g., Breland, 1974), in other characteristics the two groups did not differ, and it is doubtful whether the processes of development and of family interaction that make prediction of child from parent characteristics possible, will differ radically between twins and nontwins.

We took account of mothers' education level in the prediction analysis and, insofar as mother's education can be considered as a substitute for maternal IQ, we did at least partly control for this in assessing the influence of the home environment on the child's cognitive development. Analyzing the relation between the child's own 2-year and 9-year attributes allowed as at the same time to assess the influence the child has on his own development. The question what effect the child has on his parents is, however, not addressed in this report.

METHOD

Sample

At 2 years. The sample of the original study consisted of 46 sets of same-sex male twins (17 monozygotic [MZ], 29 dizygotic [DZ]) and 44 male singletons, a total of 136 boys. Mean age was 32.4 months, range 25–35 months.

Twins were located through the birth registers of the local hospitals and they represent almost the total male twin population born during 1969 and 1970 in a Canadian city. The singleton controls at age 2 were recruited via City Health Clinics from two-parent families and were matched pairwise with the twins for age and SES.

Both groups contained one-third middle class and two-thirds working class families (all white), as assessed by father's occupation (Blishen, 1967). The sample was thus reasonably representative of white North American families from the point of view of social class, but it contained a preponderance of twins.

At 9 years.   Because of their unique situation and special interest, only the twins of the sample received the full follow-up treatment. The singletons of the original investigation were followed up to a limited extent, when they were 6–7 years old, but these results will not be reported here.

Of the 46 original twin families, 35 participated fully in the investigation and 37 took part in the follow-up by means of teacher ratings and examination of school records. Formal consent in writing was obtained from participating families.

The sample consisted of 15 MZ and 22 DZ pairs. The mean age of the twins was 9 years 6 months, and the range 8 years 5 months to 10 years 8 months. (MZ mean: 9 yrs. 8 mths; DZ mean: 9 yrs. 5 mths.)

We ran an analysis on the seven most important 2-year variables to see whether "drop-outs" differed significantly from participating twins, and found that this was, indeed, the case. In particular, the participants were rated as more mature in their speech than the drop-outs at age 2 ($p < .01$) and their mothers' education level was higher ($p < .05$). Not only did mothers with lower education level and whose children were less cognitively advanced (as judged by speech maturity) tend to refuse participation more, but we were also less successful in reaching them, probably because their family situation was more unstable.

The loss of the drop-outs did change the nature of the twin

sample somewhat. If the drop-outs had been included, the means of the twins' cognitive ability and achievement measures would very likely have been depressed, but it is doubtful whether prediction would have been affected materially.

Procedures at 2 Years

The 2-year investigation focused on the social characteristics of attachment, independence, compliance and internalized standards, plus speech facility, studied in the context of parent-child interaction, as well as in relation to genetic factors.

The methods are described in detail in Lytton (1980). Observations of unstructured interactions between mothers, father and children in the home, coded in detail, yielded summary behavior counts. Mothers were asked to write a "diary" account of all events involving the children within a 24-hour period and they were given a standard interview. Based on the combined evidence of the observations, the "diary" and specified interview questions, the children were rated on the target characteristics and the mothers on their child-rearing practices and attitudes, e.g., consistency in enforcing rules, encouragement of independence, warmth. The median interrater reliability for mother ratings was .80 and for child ratings .67. The Peabody Picture Vocabulary Test (PPVT) which has acceptable reliability and validity (Dunn, 1965), was also administered to the children.

Procedures at 9 Years

Home-based assessments. The purpose of the home-based assessments was to obtain a) measures on the same social characteristics of the children that had been assessed at age 2 (see above), and b) measures of parents' current child-rearing practices.

A semi-structured interview was conducted concerning mothers' perceptions of their children's personality characterisitcs and mothers' attitudes and practices in relation to child-rearing. The interview was based on the interview which had been given to mothers at the time of the 2-year study, but some questions were modified to take account of changed expectations for the older age group. The rater-interviewer assigned a score for a given trait, based on the responses to all questions related to this trait. Interrate reliabilities, established by having a second rater rate six protocols, had a median of .88, with only two falling below .70.

Factor analyses were carried out on child and mother traits at age 2 and age 9 in order to achieve some data reduction. It was hoped that a few summary factors would describe the underlying structures of this domain more clearly, and that relationships among these factors would emerge more strongly than among individual variables.

The factor analyses produced some summary factors that were conceptually equivalent and that correlated across the two ages (good social functioning for the child and optimal approach for the mother). In view of this and the identical definition of the traits at the two ages we have some evidence that the measures at 2 and at 9 tapped equivalent underlying dimensions.

During the same home visit each parent was asked to complete Rutter's Children's Behavior Questionnaire (CBQ), which is a screening test for psychological maladjustment, with parallel forms for parents and teachers. Its reliabilitiy and validity (Rutter, Tizard & Whitmore, 1970) are satisfactory. Individual items are added up to form a total Maladjustment score, as well as a Neurotic subscore and an Antisocial subscore.

School-based assessments. The purpose of the school-based assessments was to secure teachers' ratings for the child social characteristics under study and to assess the children's cognitive competence and social adjustment at school.

Classroom teachers were asked to complete a Child Rating Scale of 28 items. The scale was devised to measure the same child behaviors that were rated from the parent interview, but in relation to the school situation, as well as the child's maturity of speech. These ratings were entered into the factor analysis of child traits at age 9.

The children were tested individually by a trained tester. They were given the Crichton Vocabulary Scale (CVS) and the Raven's Coloured Progressive Matrices (CPM) to test their verbal and nonverbal abilities. To measure academic achievement, the scales of the Peabody Individual Achievement Test (PIAT) were administered. All three tests are well-established and have good reliability and validity (Dunn & Markwardt, 1970; Raven, Court & Raven, 1977).

RESULTS

Overview of Prediction Analyses

Fathers' earlier attitudes and practices were correlated with the children's 9-year characteristics, but since the relationships were generally weaker than those for mother, these data will not be presented here.

The child's 9-year characteristics were predicted from both child and mother variables by multiple regression analyses. The prediction analysis assesses how well, say, the child's cognitive competence at age 9 could be predicted from what was already known about the child at age 2. Three waves of *mother variables* were entered as predictors in this stepwise multiple regression analysis at three successive steps, each wave of variables being derived from a successive point in time. The waves were: 1) the demographic context factor of mother's education level; 2) biological pregnancy and perinatal factors known to affect the child's mental development; and 3) mother's child-rearing practices when the child was 2, expressed as factor scores.

A parallel analysis demonstrated how well the child's own characteristics up to age 2, plus mother's education, predicted 9-year cognitive competence. Mother's education was included here because it comprises environmental and genetic aspects of the child's life (cf. Scarr, 1985, for a demonstration of the genetic content of the "mother education" variable).

The child's 9-year social characteristics were predicted in separate analyses from mother's practices and attitudes when the child was 2, rated individually. We used twin pair means as the

unit of analysis, since individual twins' scores are often highly
correlated with each other and entering each twin's score separately amount almost to entering the same score twice.

TABLE I
Three-Wave Prediction of Cognitive Competence
from Mother Variables

	Twin Pair Means (n = 34 pairs)		
Predictors	Multiple R^2	% of Variance explained	Simple r
1) Mother's Education	.194**	19.4	.440
2) Pregnancy Information			
Toxemia	.266**	7.2	.306
3) Mother Characteristics—Child aged 2			
FAC3: Expedience in discipline	.283*		.170
FAC1: Positive affective & cognitive		1.8	
approach vs. physical punishment	.284*		.093
R^2 adjusted for shrinkage	.193		
Total		28.4	

*$p<.05$, **$p<.01$

Cognitive Abilities

Prediction from mother's characteristics. The following explanation
will help readers unfamiliar with multiple regression to interpret
Table I. How well each predictor predicts the criterion is expressed
by the amount of the variance explained or accounted for. The
multiple R^2 in the first line tells us what proportion of the variance
in the criterion (Cognitive Competence) is explained by the first
predictor (mother's education), and thus indicates how well
mother's education predicts Cognitive Competence. The multiple
R^2 at each subsequent step indicates how much of the variance in
the criterion is explained by the predictor at that step, *plus all
previous predictors.* The "percent of variance explained" column

transforms the proportions of the R^2 to percent (proportion $\times$ 100), and at each step shows how much *additional* variance in the criterion is explained by a predictor or group of predictors, over and above the variance explained by the previous predictors. Thus, the two variables summarizing mother's characteristics at child's age 2, together account for 1.8% of the variance of cognitive competence, over and above the variance explained by mother's education and toxemia.

The "simple r" column shows the independent correlations of each predictor with the criterion. These correlations do not take account of other predictors and they therefore indicate the relative strength of the independent prediction of each predictor.

Since Total IQ (the average of the verbal and nonverbal scales) and the total of the achievement tests scores at age 9 were highly intercorrelated, we added the two percentiles together to form the composite variable "Cognitive Competence". The three-wave prediction of Cognitive Competence from mother's characteristics, when the child was 2, is shown in Table I. Mother's education is a summary variable that both reflects genetic characteristics that she transmits to the child (cf. Scarr, 1985) and sums up the general environment that she provides for him, the most important ingredient of which is doubtless appropriate cognitive stimulation. This is obviously the most substantial factor in determining the child's cognitive ability, i.e., higher education of the mother goes with greater cognitive competence in the child. That toxemia during pregnancy increased the child's ability may be surprising, but this finding has also been reported in some other investigations (e.g., Broman, Nichols, & Kennedy, 1975).

Table I displays two factors representing mother's 2-year child-rearing practices that made some contribution to predicting cognitive competence. Factor 3 combines the use of psychological punishment (i.e., criticism and temporary withdrawal of love) with the use of material rewards, and we called it "expedience in discipline". Factor 1 describes a positive cognitive and affective approach by mother, including the use of reasoning and of praise and the encouragement of independence, coupled with the absence of physical punishment. Once we have allowed for the influence of mother's education and the pregnancy condition, mother's ways of interacting with the 2-year-old child, as expressed by the factors, play only a very small role in determining the child's overall ability at 9, as can be seen in Table I. These personal ways of treating the child and of socializing him into the social world at age 2 (the degree of cognitive stimulation was not included here) do not seem to extend their influence to his cognitive ability at age 9. Mother's current child-rearing practices, at age 9 (not shown here), however, had a greater impact and explained an additional 25% of the variance of cognitive competence, the most important factors being the fostering of independence and strict standards, coupled with an appreciation of the child's worth.

Since all the maternal characteristics impinging on the child by age 2 that we measured, accounted only for 28% of the variance, the prediction of cognitive competence from mother's earlier characteristics is relatively poor, and we must conclude, therefore, that their influence, apart from that of mother's education, is rather small.

The boys' speech at 9 was rated by teachers for clarity of articulation and coherence of utterance and, although we did not include this rating of "speech maturity" in the variable "Cognitive Competence", it is obviously related to it and is an aspect of the child's cognitive ability overall. Though mother's education level did not relate significantly to speech maturity at 9, some of mother's child-rearing attitudes and practices at age 2 were found to play a facilitative role in its development; this was the case particularly for her warmth ($r = .33$) and the amount of time that she spent playing with her son ($r = .42$). These maternal characteristics therefore fostered the child's speech development.

Prediction from child characteristics. In sharp contrast to the poor prediction from mother's characteristics, however, all that we know about the child himself by age 2 predicts his cognitive ability at 9 very well (see Table II). As noted earlier, we included among these variables mother's education level, since it encompasses long-lasting genetic and contextual aspects of the child's life, although it is not strictly speaking a child characteristic. Apart from this last

TABLE II
Three-Wave Prediction of Cognitive Competence
from Child Variables

| Predictors | Twin Pair Means (n = 34 pairs) | | |
	Multiple R^2	% of Variance explained	Simple r
1) Mother's Education	.194**[a]	19.4	.440
2) Birth Information			
Birth Weight	.205*		.198
Total Stress Index	.261*	6.7	−.054
3) 2-Year Characteristics			
Vocabulary IQ	.536**[a]	27.5	.711
Compliance	.599**[a]		.386
Independence	.624**		.078
		9.0	
Speech Maturity	.625**		.493
Attachment	.626**		−.227
R^2 adjusted for shrinkage	.510		
Total		62.6	

NOTE: "Total Stress Index" is the number of stresses out of the following six which the child displayed: Interbirth Time Stress, Apgar Stress, Gestational Age Stress, Birth Weight Stress, Respiratory Distress Syndrome, Bilirubin Level Stress.

[a]Increment in R^2 significant ($p<.05$).
*$p<.05$, **$p<.01$.

effect, the variable that has by far the greatest influence on the child's later cognitive ability is the level of vocabulary knowledge that he has acquired by age 2, which explains 27% of the variance of cognitive competence. The 2-year-old's maturity of speech (clarity and completeness of utterances) also predicts later ability moderately well, but all the social characteristics at age 2 together do not add appreciably to the prediction of the 9-year-old's cognitive competence (about 9%), and their influence is therefore hardly stronger than that of mother's social practices when he was 2. The fact that all the information that we have about the 2-year-old explains 62.6% of the variance of the 9-year-old's cognitive competence arises mainly from the great influence that the child's own early cognitive characteristics exert on his development. His current social characteristics (e.g., internalized conscience, independence, peer relations at age 9), on the other hand, seem to have only a relatively small influence and explain only an additional 13% of the variance of cognitive competence.

Social Characteristics

Prediction from mother's characteristics.   Let us first discuss the relation between past maternal child-rearing attitudes and the child's social characteristics at age 9. The child's social attributes were assessed by teacher ratings and ratings based on interviews with mothers. These ratings, like those for maternal characteristics (see above), were submitted to a factor analysis in which a maladjustment

TABLE III

Multiple Regression Prediction of 9-Year Child Good Social Functioning (Factor) from Maternal Characteristics (Child's Age 2)

Twin Pair Means (n = 34 pairs)		
Criterion:	Good social functioning (Factor)	
Predictors	Multiple R^2	Simple r
Psychological Punishment	.160*[a]	.400
Warmth	.282**[a]	.386
Support Dependence	.330**	.177
Physical Punishment	.356*	−.274
Reasoning	.397*	.084
Restrictiveness	.419*	−.194
Encourage Mature Action	.433*	.065
Consistency of Enforcement	.446*	−.019
R^2 corrected for shrinkage	.273	

NOTE: [a]Increment in R^2 significant ($p < .05$)
   *$p < .05$, **$p < .01$.

score, derived from the Child Behavior Questionnaire, was also included. The factor that is of interest here is one that denotes good social functioning, as perceived by mother, and it is marked by high independence, conscience (i.e., internalized moral orientation) and compliance, and, at the opposite pole, by low dependence on teacher and low maladjustment. This is the factor best predicted by the earlier maternal child-rearing practices and the prediction is shown in Table III. The maternal variables that are most important in predicting the child's good social functioning, and that therefore seem to influence it most, are mother's use of psychological punishment (criticism and temporary withdrawal of love) and her warmth. Mother's current, 9-year, positive affective and cognitive approach to the child was also found to relate well to, and therefore, by inference, to foster his good social functioning.

The individual ratings of conscience and of compliance were predicted to a similar extent by mother's 2-year child-rearing attitudes. Warmth, psychological punishment *and* rewards (praise and approval) and the amount of play with the child were particularly strong predictors of these variables. It will be noted that psychological punishment facilitate good social functioning as well as psychological rewards did, and in the long term, therefore, it appears that disapproval of undesirable acts—presumably, so long as it does not deteriorate into constant nagging—has beneficial effects. Physical punishment, on the other hand, had the opposite effect (it impaired good social functioning), although the effect was weaker. The overall prediction of these aspects of good social functioning was quite good and the amount of variance explained (45% in the summary factor shown in the Table, 56% in conscience and 54% in compliance) exceeded that accounted for in cognitive competence by the three waves of maternal characteristics.

The extent to which social maladjustment was predictable was more modest (a total of 34% of variance explained). The 2-year maternal characteristics here acted in a direction opposite to that for good social functioning: maladjustment was predicted by a lack of warmth, by lack of psychological punishment and by the frequent use of physical punishment. The most notable predictor was absence of warmth in the mother. It may well be that a certain lack of warmth in the mother, noted when the child was 2, but no doubt continuing, exerted a deleterious effect on his adjustment over time. On the other hand, it is possible that the child exhibited signs of maladaptive and undesirable behaviour even at the age of 2, which would have led mother to be less affectionate toward him. The present analysis does not allow us to decide between these alternatives.

Prediction from child characteristics.   An attempt was made to predict each of the child's social characteristics, as well as the summary factors, from the three waves of child predictors that so successfully predicted his cognitive competence. However, none of these predictions, even that of the relatively best predicted characteristic, compliance, reached significance overall. The prediction of the child's social characteristics from his own earlier attributes, therefore, in contrast to the prediction of cognitive competence, seems less fruitful.

CONCLUSIONS

Cognitive ability at age 9, we found, could be predicted fairly well from mother's education level. The fact that this summary contextual variable encompasses enduring genetic and environmental aspects of the child's life explains why it so influential. On the other hand, mother's past socialization practices made only a minimal contribution to the prediction of cognitive competence. What was known about the child himself by age 2, however, predicted his 9-year cognitive ability very well, and this good prediction was in large measure attributable to the predictive power of the vocabulary IQ. The child's early social characteristics by themselves, on the other hand, did not add much to the prediction of later cognitive competence.

The picture for the child's characteristics at age 9 is rather different. These attributes were very poorly predicted from the child's own earlier characteristics. On the other hand, mother's earlier socialization practices were quite effective predictors of the general factor of good social functioning at age 9, and of some of its individual manifestations, such as conscience and compliance. The particular maternal characteristics at age 2 that proved to be significantly related to good social functioning at 9 were her warmth, her use of psychological rewards and punishments, and the amount of play with the child. Conversely, the absence of these characteristics predicted social maladjustment, though the prediction was weaker.

What are the reasons for the differences in prediction for cognitive ability and social characteristics? We can offer some speculative comments about these. Cognitive competence, it seems to us, is more under the influence of the child's own disposition and the level of environmental stimulation in the home, which is, no doubt, reflected in mother's education level. However, mother's earlier personal attitudes and the nature of disciplinary interactions with the child do not exert a strong influence on cognitive competence in the long term.

For the child's social characteristics the situation is reversed: for these the child's own disposition and the general context of mother's education level are less important; rather, they are more influenced by the processes of mother-child interaction, as expressed by her socialization practices at age 2, whose influence carries over right up to age 9. Over and above this, however, mother's current positive approach also promotes the child's good social functioning.

References

Blishen, B.R. (1967). A socio-economic index for occupations in Canada, *Canadian Rev. of Social. and Anthrop.*, **4**, 41–53.

Breland, H.M. (1974). Birth order, family configuration and verbal achievement, *Child Development*, **45**, 1011–19.

Broman, S.H., P.L. Nichols, & Kennedy, W.A. (1975). *Preschool IQ: Prenatal and early developmental correlates*, Hillsdale, N.J.: Erlbaum.

Clarke-Stewart, K.A., & Apfel, N. (1978). Evaluating parental effects on child development, *Rev. of Res. in Education*, **6**, 49–119.

Dunn, L.M. (1965). *Peabody Picture Vocabulary Test Manual*, Circle Pines, Minn.: American Guidance Service, Inc.

Dunn, L.M., & F.C. Markwardt, (1970). *Peabody Individual Achievement Test Manual*, Circle Pines, Minn.: American Guidance Service, Inc.

Lytton, H. (1980). *Parent-child interaction: The socialization process observed in twin and singleton families*, NY: Plenum.

McCall, R.B., Applebaum, M.I., & Hogarty, P.S. (1973). Developmental changes in mental performance, *Mons. of the Soc. for Res. in Child Development*, **38**, (3, Serial No. 150).

Raven, J.C., Court, J.H., & Raven, C. (1977). *Manual for Raven's Progressive Matrices and Vocabulary Scales (Revised)*, London: H.K. Lewis & Co.

Rutter, M. (1985). Family and school influences on cognitive development, *Journal of Child Psychology and Psychiatry*, **26**, 683–704.

Rutter, M., Tizard, J., & Whitmore, K. (1970). *Education, health and behavior*, London: Longman.

Scarr, S. (1985). Constructing psychology: Making facts and fables for out times, *American Psychology*, **40**, 499–512.

Parent training, home environment, and early childhood development: A long-term follow-up study[1]

EDWARD E. GOTTS[2]

Huntington State Hospital
Huntington, West Virginia

Families and children who participated in a primary prevention experiment called Home Oriented Preschool Education (HOPE) were assessed during a follow-up study approximately ten years following the experiment. Home environment and social class were assessed for families, and children's ability and achievement test scores and grade point averages were obtained from school records. Home environment was shown to be only modestly related to social class and to account for significant amounts of variance in children's academic and intellectual progress. Home environment appeared, moreover, to be affected favorably by the HOPE experiment when comparing randomly assigned groups of experimental and control families. Discussion focuses on the value of measuring home environment in studies of early childhood development.

BACKGROUND

In the years 1968–1971, a now widely-cited experiment, the Home-Oriented Preschool Education (HOPE) Program, was conducted in the eastern United States. HOPE was designed (1966–1968) by the Appalachia Educational Laboratory (AEL), an educational research and development agency, in response to its

---

1. This study was supported by various grants and contracts from the National Institute of Education and administered through the Appalachia Educational Laboratory, Inc., whose support and encouragement are gratefully acknowledged.

2. Requests for reprints should be sent to the Author:
c/o AEL, Inc.
P.O. Box 1348
Charleston, WV 25325

findings of the early childhood development needs of families and preschool children (3–5 year olds) in its seven-state region (Alabama, Kentucky, Ohio, Pennsylvania, Tennessee, Virginia, and West Virginia). A comprehensive review and follow-up study of the experiment was conducted from 1978–1982 (Gotts, 1983).

For purposes of understanding the present study, it is necessary as background to consider the original experimental design, sampling procedure, and parent training provided. These are summarized below.

A four-country area in Central Appalachia (southern West Virginia) was the study site, an area historically isolated. Residents of the study area lived in small cities (20,000 population maximum), towns, villages, and isolated rural locations. Although coal mining is the principal industry of the region, a wide range of occupations is found among the population. Most social class levels are present in the population, although their median is below the national average.

A grid-like matrix was first superimposed on detailed maps of the study's geographic area. A coded designation was assigned to each cell of the grid. A sample of these coded designations was next randomly selected, and locally hired and trained staff went out to contact all families of preschool children within each of the geographic sites designated by this random procedure.

All of the study families thus located and contacted were formally invited to participate with their children in HOPE. They were told that, if they agreed to participate, they were assured of a place in the program. They were further told: (a) there would be three variations of HOPE; (b) they would be assigned to one of these; (c) the selection process for the three variations would be determined by chance (i.e., by random selection); (d) thus, making it impossible to know in advance which variation they would receive. Over 90 percent of the families agreed to participate and were randomly assigned to the conditions as they had been told. In addition to these families, another comparable sample was selected from outside the site. The reason for this latter sample will become apparent as the treatment and control group conditions are considered next.

All families in the treatment communities received a daily television series, AROUND THE BEND, while those of the outside control group did not receive the broadcast signal. AROUND THE BEND appealed to three-through five-year-old children by presenting learning activities in an entertaining, rurally-oriented format. Within the treatment site, some families received only the television portion of the program (TV-only group). In contrast to the outside control families, the TV-only families served as a within-community control group. The remaining two groups of families received weekly visits from a paraprofessional home visitor (HV) who (a) provided them with coordinated print materials matching the television series, (b) assisted them to individualize home learning activities for their children, and (c) became friends and confidantes who helped with a variety of child development and family support issues. The children from one of the two home visited groups were further assigned to receive weekly one-half day experiences with other children in a mobile classroom van staffed by a teacher and an aide. The foregoing four groups were identified, respectively, as (1) outside control, (2) TV-only or community control, (3) TV-HV, and (4) TV-HV-Group Experience or "Package".

Families and children participated in this early childhood alternative to traditional kindergarten for from one to three years, depending upon the child's age at the time of initial entry. Following the program, the groups all proceeded into the years of schooling without being identified in their local school as HOPE participants. Unlike participants in some other widely-known preschool programs, this fact permitted them to be received and treated by the schools in accordance with their respective characteristics rather than as representatives of a particular program or movement.

Ten years later on the average, families and children from the latter three groups (i.e., TV-only, TV-HV, and Package) were located through a thorough search of the four-country HOPE area. Because families and children of the outside control group had experienced different schools and were, thus, no longer comparable, no attempt was made to locate them for this follow-up effort.

For purposes of the analyses to be reported later below, the TV-HV and Package groups were combined in recognition of their common experience of receiving home visitation. Prior comparisons of these two groups made immediately after their HOPE participation showed that they performed similarly on many early childhood tests and could reasonably be combined (see Gotts, 1983). In this manner, the original design could be simplified to a two group comparison and contrast: community control (TV only) versus home visited (TV-HV plus Package).

Families and children in the foregoing two groups had had up to ten years experience in and with the same schools in the identified communities. By means of random assignment, the two groups had been established initially as not different from each other in terms of social class and other demographic characteristics—and initial measurements of social class showed them to be comparable. The respect in which the parents differed, on the other hand, is that some had received one to three years of home visitation when their children were preschoolers, while the remainder had received TV only. This experimentally-arranged difference ten-years prior to the follow-up study lent itself to an analysis of ways in which (1) the parents might now be different, (2) the children might have experienced differing school outcomes, and (3) any parent and children differences might be related and traceable to the experimental treatment of home visitation.

HOME ENVIRONMENT AND DEVELOPMENT

Particularly since the work of Coleman (1966), the importance of family background to school achievement has been recognized and increasingly studied. Often family social class, as represented by scales of family income, education, and occupational level—and by combinations of these—has been used as the primary index of family background. A historical review of the study of social class is presented as a series of analytic models by Walberg and Marjoribanks (1976). Social class is, unfortunately, a fairly broad, remote, and indirect indicator of the particular ways in which family background is expressed toward and experienced by children. For this reason it has become increasingly common to hear social class referred to as a "proxy variable," (Dolan, 1983), i.e., social class stands for a complex reality that it neither measures nor expresses directly. Social class is, nevertheless, sufficiently correlated with the complex reality of family background to have served as a useful statistical and classificatory substitute for it. Despite a positive and consistently found empirical relation between social class and family background, dissatisfaction has been expressed with this proxy variable because (1) it does not fully represent the reality of family environment (Walberg and Marjoribanks, 1976) and (2) social class is a static index that is not easily altered by the usual forms of social-educational intervention, thus rendering it of limited practical benefit to researchers seeking to improve children's intellectual and educational performance. Specifically, social class indicates only what parents are like rather than the things they do that may affect their children's performance (Dolan, 1983).

In response to the foregoing types of concerns, a measure of home environment processes was developed through collaborative efforts of investigators at the University of Chicago (Dave, 1963; Wolf, 1964). Items were administered by interview to mothers. Item content concerned what parents do with and for their children outside of school (i.e., at home and in the community) that may stimulate their learning and development. Examples of specific areas represented were: verbal interaction in the home, availability of learning materials and supplies, the parent as a role model of a "learner," and intellectual aspirations for the child. While the interview does not measure these process variables directly (Longstreth, 1978), it elicits parents' self reports about them in sufficiently specific detail to make it reasonable to assume a positive relationship between the actual home environment and the replies given (Trotman, 1978).

Parent responses to the home environment scale (H.E.S.) questions were rated using standard instructions and scales for each item. With the H.E.S. items summed to form an overall scale, its internal consistency reliability coefficient was around .90 in various studies (Trotman, 1977). The H.E.S. was substantially correlated with both ability and achievement, with these relationships exceeding those usually found between social class and either ability or achievement (Dave, 1963; Wolf, 1964). The foregoing and later studies using the H.E.S. and similar procedures have suggested that interview measures of home environment process may be better predictors of children's intellectual competence and achievement than are traditional measures of social class (Trotman, 1977; Walberg & Marjoribanks, 1976).

Staff of AEL were impressed by the results obtained with the original H.E.S. Accordingly when they began planning in 1977 to perform a long term follow-up study of HOPE program participants, they decided to prepare an adaptation of the H.E.S., using the original work of Dave (1963) and Wolf (1964) as a prototype.

In commencing this work it was noted that some overlap existed between the content of the H.E.S. and of Interview I of a study protocol developed somewhat earlier for use at the Fels Research Institute for the Study of Human Development. The Fels' instrument sampled parents' intellectual attainment (achievement) value, evaluation (expectation) of the child's competence, satisfaction-dissatisfaction with the child's performance, minimal standards, instigation of intellectual activities, participation in the child's activities, and affective reactions (Positive-negative) to the child's intellectual achievement behaviours (Crandall, Dewey, Katkovsky & Preston, 1964). AEL staff planned to use the Fels' measures also, so found it necessary to exclude certain Fels' items from their H.E.S. adaptation in order to eliminate potentially troublesome overlaps. Some content areas originally appearing in both lines of work were retained and scored in the H.E.S. only.

The resulting AEL H.E.S. consisted of interview questions from which ratings were made of 18 aspects of the home environment. These are listed in Table I.

Based on a small sample, inter-rater agreement for the 18-item scale's total score was .91 (n = 39). The internal consistency (alpha coefficient) of the AEL H.E.S. was .76 for the total sample (n = 226). Total score for the H.E.S. was a normally distributed

TABLE I
Aspects Rated in AEL Home Environment Scale (H.E.S.)

1. Number of outside activities parent encourages (and child engages in)
2. Number of special lessons/training provided child.
3. Number of classes parent took/taking and how doing.
4. Number of opportunities for child to take trips (and learn).
5. Extent of parents' observable reading.
6. Number of newspapers and magazines in home.
7. Possession and use of library card.
8. Presence and use of dictionary in home.
9. Presence and use of encyclopedia in home.
10. Extent TV viewing regulated and used educationally.
11. Time family is together and interacting verbally.
12. Amount and quality of father's interaction with child.
13. Amount of assistance with homework.
14. How far parent wants child to go in school.
15. How far parent expects child to go in school.
16. Least amount of schooling parents say child must have.
17. Education required for level occupation parent desires for child.
18. Extent parent models participation in outside activities/hobbies.

variable. By definition, with each rating running from *1* to *7*, scale scores could range from a minimum of *18* to a maximum of *126*, with higher scores representing more favorable home environments. The defined mid-point of the scale is *72*. The actual mean H.E.S. score for the HOPE follow-up study sample was *78.77*— slightly above the scale's defined mean. On the average there was relative absence of tendencies either for parents to give answers suggesting self-report stereotypy or for raters to rate the interview records in ways indicating halo effect; consequently H.E.S. scores were neither near the minimum nor maximum possible (actual range 40–106). Further discussion of the H.E.S. appears below in the Findings section.

Finally, to get a further sense of the meaning of the AEL version of the H.E.S., correlations were computed between the individual items and the total score. The following items (See Table I) best defined the scale's meaning: *4* (.51), *5* (.49), *6* (.46), *14* (.45), *1* (.44), and *18* (.41). It is noteworthy that only one of these items (i.e., item *14*) deals in a more obvious manner with schooling as such. The items that related most weakly to the total score were: *16* (.13), *17* (.15), *7* (.17), *10* (.25), and *13* (.25), which as a group would appear to relate more obviously to achievement. Considering together the most strongly and weakly related item groups, the meaning of the H.E.S. appears to be more subtle than obvious relative to the linkage between home environment and intellectual pursuits. The items not listed above were correlated with the H.E.S. at levels intermediate to those already cited.

PROCEDURES

All parents were interviewed in their own homes by local interviewers from their geographic area. Interviewers were not aware of whether those interviewed had been in the experimental or control group. In fact, the interviewers were not aware that the participants were differentiated into groups. Arbitrary ID numbers had been assigned randomly to cases to prevent inadvertent discovery of group membership within the sample. All interviews were recorded onto audio cassettes using battery operated recorders. Subsequently they were transcribed verbatim in another location. Next the transcripts and tapes were reviewed coordinately by another staff member for accuracy. Following this the typed transcripts were sent to a third location for rating by a doctoral level professional who was otherwise unrelated to the study and remained uninformed of group membership or other particulars of the study. None of the foregoing parties was aware of the academic records or achievement test results of the children whose parents were interviewed, so the potential for experimenter bias (see Wolff, 1978) was essentially eliminated by the precautions employed.

The items of the H.E.S. appeared in Parts I and IV of an interview sequence called the "Direct Parent Interview" by AEL. It was so designated because it involved the parent directly in self reflection and report. Part VII of this same interview included questions regarding family social class. These were administered and the answers transcribed and coded as previously described. Social class was coded using the Hollingshead two-factor index

(Hollingshead and Redlich, 1958). Because the Hollingshead index is coded with a low score meaning high status, the social class scores were arithmetically reflected in order to make a high score signify high status and, thus, to simplify interpretation and reporting.

Three years before the follow-up study began, a preliminary search was made in local school records of the four county system to determine how many children could be located. Over 200 families which had remained in their original communities (i.e., near a particular elementary or junior high school) were found at that time. Data from their school cumulative records were collected and coded then; they were updated three years later. Additional families were located in 1977–78, as the follow-up study got under way. No exhaustive attempt was made to locate all families, however, because resources available for this in-depth and costly-to-perform study were sufficient for inclusion of only about 225 complete family cases. When this cost-imposed limit had been reached, no further families were contacted.

As noted earlier, the experimental and control groups initially did not differ in social class. This was rechecked to see if either sample attrition or the method used to limit the size of the follow-up sample might have altered the initial social class-neutral division of experimental (E) and control (C) groups. The correlation between social class and group membership (E vs. C) was .15 (n = 226), a significant (p < .05, but p > .01) yet very modest positive relationship—i.e., experimental families were more likely to be of higher social class. Social class accounted for only slightly over two percent of the variance in group membership.

FINDINGS

First, it is interesting to note the significant but relatively unimpressive relationship between social class and home environment scores (r = .40, n = 195, p < .01). I say "unimpressive" not because this correlation is small—it is not—but because in prior discussions in the literature, social class and home environment

F

have been presented as being two different ways of looking at a fundamentally similar underlying reality, yet the fact is that their similarity is fairly modest, accounting for just sixteen percent or about one-sixth of the variance of each. Thus, social class cannot be considered a satisfactory proxy variable for what is measured by the H.E.S.

It is, then, further instructive to examine the relationship of social class and home environment, respectively, to various measures of children's intellectual competence and accomplishment and parents' orientation toward schooling. These relations are summarized in Table II as follows.

In interpreting Table II it is necessary to know that the ability and achievement test scores and the teacher grades used were all computed means from records beginning in preschool years and continuing through the highest grade level or testing period for which records were available. That is, the variables used are based on multiple occasions and are unusually stable estimates of ability and achievement.

TABLE II

Correlations of Social Class and Home Environment with Intellectual/ Achievement Measures

	Social Class		Home Environment	
	Exper.	Control	Exper.	Control
Achievement Test Mean	.37	.36	.30	.39
Mean Teacher Grades	.31	.48[2]	.26	.55[5]
Ability Test Mean	.34	.54[3]	.39	.42
Parents' Academic Orientation	.26	.29[1]	.45	.50
Home Environment	.33	.49[4]		

[1] $p < .05$; all other correlations in table $p < .01$, with n's for Experimental and Control groups, respectively, of 159 and 51.
[2] difference between correlations $z = 1.224$, $p < .12$
[3] difference between correlations $z = 1.515$, $p < .07$
[4] difference between correlations $z = 1.169$, $p < .13$
[5] difference between correlations $z = 2.133$, $p < .02$

Whereas social class and home environment did not appear to measure the same thing, they were about equally effective in predicting children's achievement and ability. The H.E.S., on the other hand, related more strongly to an interview measure of parents' academic orientation, as assessed by a test of the significance of the difference between two correlations ($z = 2.38$, $p<.01$). As might be expected from the foregoing, social class and home environment worked in a complementary manner with one another when both were used in regression equations predicting how well children were doing in school. For example, when attempts were made to predict a special composite score of children's functioning in school, both social class and home environment were entered in the equation along with the treatment effect and other variables.

Examination of differences between correlations for the Experimental and Control groups (Table II), using the z-transformation method, produced four interesting and consistent findings that point in common directions: participation in the home enrichment program appeared to attenuate the effects of a child's family background on the child's performance in school and to reduce the relationship between social class and the quality of home learning environment provided. Specifically, the relationship of both social class ($p<.12$) and home environment ($p<.02$) to long-term teacher grades appeared to diminish as a result of parents' participation in a home-oriented preschool program. A similar drop is noted for the relationship between social class and the child's ability ($p<.07$). Social class had seemingly become a less powerful determinant of home environment for the Experimental group ($p<.13$). All of these findings further represent directionally similar declines within pairs of correlations that are all highly significant in both the Experimental and Control groups—i.e., reduction of highly reliable relationships.

Finally, the home environment scores of parents who had received home visitor assistance with child development (experimental group) were compared to those of the community control group after an average of about ten years. The experimental group's mean (4.14 vs. 4.11) exceeded that of the control group

$(t = 2.43,\ df = 210,\ p = .016)$, suggesting that participation in HOPE's home component may have affected the home environment favorably.

DISCUSSION

When the effect of HOPE on the favorability of home environment is considered together with the evidence that home environment relates to academic-intellectual outcome (See Table II) and that its relation to social class is too small to explain this, the composite results would suggest that HOPE affected academic-intellectual outcome in part by strengthening the home learning environment. Comparison of the classroom grades of experimental and control groups in fact confirmed that HOPE resulted in higher academic performance in the first two grades, whereas from grade three onward the groups no longer differed (Gotts, 1983). In contrast to the fading out of differences in grade point average, the overall academic careers of the experimental children were found to be more favorable when considered in terms of the probability that they failed a grade in school. Gotts (1983) found that about 25 percent of children in the control group were held back in school at least one year, while this was true for only about five percent of the experimental group $(\chi^2 = 10.350,\ p < .01)$. Further study is ongoing at this time to clarify HOPE's longer term effects on rates of graduation from high school and on participation in post-secondary education.

Other studies suggested that the HOPE treatment resulted in better coping skills in school as evidenced by both fewer depressive symptoms and higher levels of conventional adjustment in children of the treatment group (Gotts, 1983). Toward the end of the children's secondary years, HOPE parents were interviewed regarding their handling of school-family relations. Those in the experimental group had an edge in several respects over the control group in this regard.

Home environment, thus, commends itself as a measurement focus in early childhood development studies because (1) process aspects can thereby be sampled, (2) empirical relations exist between home environment measures and indicators of intellectual and academic progress, (3) home environment is susceptible of experimental change more readily than social class, (4) home environment changes can be reflected on scales like the H.E.S. in the years following program participation, i.e., they reflect not only status but are also sensitive to change, (5) home environment is more than social class, making the latter an unsatisfactory proxy for it, and (6) measures of home environment and social class are complementary to one another, leading to better prediction when used together than when social class is used alone.

Future reports on the HOPE follow-up study will examine how the H.E.S. operates in conjunction with measures of parental nurturing and affection and academic orientation to influence child outcomes.

References

Coleman, J.S., Campbell, E.Q., Hobson, C.J., McPartland, J., Mood, A.M., Weinfeld, F.D., and York, R.L. (1966). *Equality of educational opportunity*, Washington, D.C.; U.S. Government Printing Office.

Crandall, V., Dewey, R., Katkovsky, W., & Preston, A. (1964). Parents' attitudes and behaviors and grade-school children's academic achievements. *The Journal of Genetic Psychology*, **104,** 53–66.

Davè, R. (1963). *The identification and measurement of home environmental process variables related to educational achievement.* Unpublished doctoral dissertation, University of Chicago.

Dolan, L (1983). The prediction of reading achievement and self-esteem from an index of home educational environment: a study of urban elementary students. *Measurement and Evaluation in Guidance*, **16,** 86–94.

Gotts, E.E. (1983). Home-based early intervention. In A.W. Childs & G.B. Melton (Eds.), *Rural psychology* (pp. 337–48). New York: Plenum.

Hollingshead, A.B., & Redlich, F.C. (1958). *Social class and mental illness.* New York: Wiley.

Longstreth, L.E. (1978). A comment on "Race, IQ, and the middle class" by Trotman: rampant false conclusions. *Journal of Educational Psychology*, **70,** 469–72.

Trotman, F.K. (1977). Race, IQ, and the middle class. *Journal of Educational Psychology*, **69,** 266–73.

Trotman, F.K. (1978). Race, IQ, and rampant in misrepresentations: a reply. *Journal of Educational Psychology*, **70,** 478–481.

Walberg, H.J., & Marjoribanks, K. (1976). Family environment and cognitive development, Twelve analytic models, *Review of Educational Research*, **46,** 527–51.

Wolf, R.M. (1964). *The identification and measurement of home environmental process variables that are related to intelligence.* Unpublished doctoral dissertation, University of Chicago.

Wolff, J.L. (1978). Utility of socioeconomic status as a control in racial comparisons of IQ, *Journal of Educational Psychology*, **70,** 473–477.

Parental modernity and child academic competence: Toward a theory of individual and societal development

EARL S. SCHAEFER

A longitudinal study of low income mothers and infants investigated relationships among parent behaviors and characteristics and child adaptive behaviors in kindergarten. Substantial intercorrelated childrearing and educational beliefs, values, and behaviors that were labelled parental modernity were correlated with parent education and individual modernity. Childrearing beliefs, values for children, and parent behaviors during infancy and the pre-school years were significantly correlated with child academic competence and motivation. An environmental interpretation of correlations of parental modernity with child academic competence was supported by evidence of historical increases in mean intelligence levels that correspond to progress in education and technology. Parallel increases in societal modernity, individual/parental modernity, and child academic competence are integrated by a theory of individual and societal development.

Longitudinal research on correlations of parental modernity with child academic competence and an environmental interpretation of those correlations provide a basis for an analysis of relationships among concepts of societal modernity, adult individual and parental modernity, and child modernity and academic competence. A major objective of this longitudinal research was to study maternal characteristics during pregnancy and child's infancy that predict the child's academic competence at school entrance. The study was designed to contribute to cross-sectional and longitudinal research on environmental correlates of child intellectual development (Hunt, 1961) that has motivated the development of early interventions to foster child development. Yet evaluations of parent-centered interventions have often not evaluated effects upon parents but have been limited to effects of intervention on the child (Simeonson, Cooper, and Scheiner, 1982). Therefore, a second objective of this longitudinal research was to contribute to development and validation of measures of maternal characteristics that are correlated with child development.

The concept of parental modernity to describe the set of parent beliefs, values and behaviors that are correlated with child intellectual development (Schaefer & Edgerton, 1985) was suggested by research on overall individual modernity of adults in six developing nations (Inkeles & Smith, 1974). Increases during the twentieth century in mean intelligence of adults and children in the United States (Flynn, 1984; Tuddenham, 1948) that correspond to progress in education, science and technology during that period (Bell, 1973) support an environmental interpretation of correlations of parental modernity with child academic competence. Evidence of correlations between parental modernity and child development and of correspondence between development of modern society and historical increases in mean intellectual levels can be integrated by an environmental theory of societal and individual development.

RESEARCH DESIGN

The longitudinal study was designed both to study correlates of maternal attachment to the infant and to influence maternal attachment by increased mother-infant contact during the first three days after birth in the hospital and by ten home visits by paraprofessionals during the first three months of life. Although effects of the paraprofessional home visits upon maternal behavior were significant only at four months but not at twelve months postnatally, maternal socioeconomic and psychosocial characteristics had substantial correlations with maternal behavior at both four and twelve months postnatally (Siegel, Bauman, Schaefer, Saunders & Ingrams, 1980). The extensive data on maternal characteristics and behavior collected during the third trimester of pregnancy and at four and twelve months postnatally motivated a longitudinal folllow-up during the kindergarten year to investigate the stability of maternal characteristics and the predictability of child school adaptation from pregnancy, infancy, and kindergarten data on the mothers.

The sample at birth consisted of 321 low-income mothers who had received prenatal services from a local public health agency and who delivered healthy infants in a community hospital. The 269 mothers who participated in data collection at four and/or twelve months postnatally were selected as the sample for the longitudinal study, of whom 237 were interviewed during the child's kindergarten year.

Data on maternal psychosocial and socioeconomic characteristics were collected during extensive interviews during the third trimester of pregnancy, at four and twelve months postnatally, and during the child's kindergarten year at the ages of five to six years. Data on maternal behavior with the infant were collected from observations during the interview and during child care situations of bathing, dressing, and play. Data on maternal childrearing and educational beliefs. values, and behavior were also collected during interviews. Data on child adaptive behavior in kindergarten were collected from teacher ratings and from school records of grade retention or promotion at the end of kindergarten.

Measurement of maternal behavior during infancy

Methods for quantifying maternal behavior at four and twelve months postnatally were needed to achieve the goal of evaluating the effects of the hospital and home visit interventions upon maternal attachment to the infant. Guided by an interpretation of maternal attachment as affection and involvement, standard forms were developed on which observations of quantity and quality of mother-infant interaction were recorded immediately after specific child care situations of bathing, dressing and play. Ratings were completed after the home visit on an Attachment Inventory that consisted of 75 specific items that were developed from earlier observational research on maternal behavior (Schaefer, Bell & Bayley, 1959). Reliability of the observations and ratings was determined by collecting data from two observers for each home visit. The extensive data collected by the two observers were integrated by independent factor analyses of ratings on the

Attachment Inventory and of the observation data from each child care situation. Two major dimensions of maternal behavior were replicated for each method both at four and at twelve months.

Factor analyses of the Attachment Inventory ratings yielded two dimensions of Interaction/Stimulation and of Punitiveness/Irritability. An order of neighboring of correlated clusters of maternal behavior items within the positive quadrant of a two-dimensional plot consisted of a sequence of achievement press, stimulation, interaction, pleasure in mothering, and responsiveness; and within the negative quadrant a sequence of low interaction, unresponsiveness, insensitivity, irritability, and punitiveness. Although cluster scores for interaction versus low interaction and responsiveness versus unresponsiveness were highly negatively correlated, the dimension of Interaction/Stimulation was best defined by positive items and the dimension of Punitiveness/Irritability by negative items.

Factor analyses of the observations of the child care situations of bathing, dressing, and play also identified two major factors of (1) Mother-Infant Interaction and (2) Gentle, Sensitive versus Rough, Insensitive Behavior. Substantial intercorrelations of corresponding rating and observation factors and replication of factors at four and twelve months suggest that the two dimensions might be identified in other data on maternal behavior. However, scores for Interaction/Stimulation revealed higher variability, higher interrater reliability, and higher stability from four to twelve months than scores for Punitiveness/Irritability.

MEASURES OF CHILDREARING AND EDUCATIONAL BELIEFS AND VALUES

Parent attitude, belief, and value measures were collected during interviews at twelve months postnatally and during kindergarten. Parental values were collected with a version of Kohn's (1969) rank-order method that contrasted conforming values of obedience, politeness, and manners with self-directing values of independent thinking, curiosity, and imagination. Parent beliefs about child-rearing and education were collected with a Parental Modernity Inventory (Schaefer & Edgerton, 1985) that measures traditional authoritarian belief including beliefs in "absolute authority of parent and of teacher", "children are born bad and will misbehave if permitted" and "children learn passively and should be treated uniformly." and progressive, democratic beliefs that "parents should encourage expression of the child's ideas," "children learn actively," and "the aim of education is learning how to learn." This longitudinal study confirmed earlier cross-sectional findings of correlations between authoritarian beliefs and conforming values and between democratic beliefs and self-directing values for children (Schaefer & Edgerton, 1985).

PARENTAL MODERNITY IN BELIEFS, VAULES, AND BEHAVIORS

Longitudinal research on this low income sample has identified significant correlations between maternal behavior observation of Interaction/Stimulation during infancy and maternal interview reports during kindergarten of earlier age of teaching academic skills, providing educational experience in family and community, and sharing activities and talking with the child. Both the observation and interview data on maternal educational behavior with the child are significantly positively correlated with maternal democratic beliefs and self-directing values and negatively correlated with authoritarian beliefs and conforming values for children. Thus correlations among observation and interview data support the development of a concept of parental modernity in childrearing and educational beliefs, values, and behaviors.

PARENTAL MODERNITY, INDIVIDUAL MODERNITY, SOCIOECONOMIC STATUS, AND INTELLIGENCE

A syndrome of individual modernity that was replicated by Inkeles and Smith (1974) in six developing nations also included belief and value measures of efficacy, active citizenship, change valuation, education valuation, new experience valuation, and technical skill valuation. Individual modernity measures of agreement with "...granting of more autonomy and rights to those of lesser status and power, such as minority groups and women" (Inkeles and Smith, 1974, p. 109) are similar to parental modernity measures of democratic childrearing beliefs and self-directing values for children (Schaefer & Edgerton, 1985).

Both parental modernity and individual modernity are substantially correlated with education (Schaefer & Edgerton, 1985; Inkeles and Smith, 1974) and, in the kindergarten interview of this longitudinal study, are significantly correlated with one another. Both parental modernity and individual modernity measures are also correlated with receptive vocabulary and with information scores, which may be interpreted as measures of parent intelligence. The significant correlations among measures of parental modernity, individual modernity, and intelligence and the correlations of each with parent education and occupation suggest that the several measures are each indicators of the cultural or psychosocial environment of the family.

CHILD ADAPTIVE BEHAVIOR IN THE CLASSROOM

Data on child adaptive behavior in kindergarten were collected with teacher rating methods that were developed in a program of research on conceptualization, measurement and development of conceptual models for child behavior (Schaefer, 1961, 1971, 1981). Initially scales for social and emotional behavior contributed to the isolation of a two-dimensional, circumplex model for child behavior with dimensions of Extraversion versus Introversion and Considerateness versus Hostility (Schaefer, 1961). Further scale development and factor analysis identified a dimension of Task-Orientation versus Distractibility with positive scales of perseverance, attention, concentration, methodicalness, and achievement orientation and negative scales of distractibility, hyperactivity, and inappropriate talkativeness (Schaefer, 1971).

A more dynamic learning style dimension was identified from highly intercorrelated scales for Curiosity and Creativity. A goal of collecting teacher ratings of child intelligence motivated development of items for vocabulary, information, comprehension, generalization, and assimilation of ideas which were integrated by a factor of Verbal Intelligence. Items that describe child initiative and decisiveness in academic work were integrated in a dimension of Instrumental Independence.

Factor analyses of the combined scales isolated a factor of Academic Competence and replicated the initial factors of Extraversion versus Introversion and Considerateness versus Hostility. The dimension of Academic Competence was best defined by verbal intelligence but also had loadings for positive scales of curiosity/creativity, task-orientation, and independence and negative scales of apathy, inattention, dependency, distractibility, and hyperactivity. Scales with loadings on Academic Competence that describe conation or motivation also have loadings on social adjustment factors, e.g., hyperactivity and distractibility are correlated with hostility and antisocial behavior whereas apathy and inattention are correlated with withdrawal and depression.

The differention of a dimension of academic competence from two dimensions of social adjustment suggests that academic competence and social adjustment have different antecedents and correlates. The Classroom Behavior Inventory (Schaefer & Edgerton, 1979) that includes positive scales for verbal intelligence, curiosity/creativity, independence, task-orientation, considerateness,· and extroversion and negative scales for dependency, distractibility, hostility, and introversion provides a reliable and valid method for collecting teacher ratings (Schaefer, 1981). A three-dimensional, spherical model for child behavior developed from factor analysis and multidemensional scaling analysis reveals a unified model for academic competence and social adjustment that facilitates integration of studies of child behavior from the fields of child development, educational psychology, abnormal child psychology, and child psychiatry. For example, current diagnostic concepts of conduct disorder, anxiety disorder, attention deficit disorder with hyperactivity, and mental retardation can be identified with different sectors of the spherical model. Morever, conceptualization of positive, adaptive behaviors may contribute to development of positive goals in programs designed to promote development and to prevent or treat pathology.

CORRELATIONS OF PARENTAL INDIVIDUAL MODERNITY WITH CHILD ACADEMIC COMPETENCE

Major factors of mother-infant interaction that were identified from observations and ratings at four and twelve months postnatally were significantly correlated with teacher ratings of child behavior during the spring of the kindergarten year. Significant correlations were found of kindergarten teacher ratings of verbal intelligence and curiosity/creativity with both observation and rating factors of mother-infant interaction at four months, but with higher correlations at twelve months postnatally. Factors derived from ratings of maternal behavior at the end of the home visit on the Attachment Inventory yielded higher correlations with child academic competence in kindergarten than factors derived from extensive observations of child care during bathing, dressing, and play. Attachment Inventory scales of achievement press, stimulation, and interaction were consistently significantly correlated with teacher ratings of verbal intelligence and curiosity/creativity with somewhat lower correlations with scales of independence and task-orientation.

Further evidence of the predictive validity of ratings of maternal behavior during infancy was found in correlations with child retention versus promotion at the end of the kindergarten year. Both the four and twelve month ratings of high levels of mother-infant interaction were significantly correlated with child promotion to first grade. Sums of all observation and rating items at four and twelve months that describe mother's responsiveness and verbal responsiveness to the infant had the highest correlations with promotion at the end of kindergarten, with the correlation for total responsiveness $(r = .39, p < .001)$ as high as the correlation of promotion with teacher ratings of child's verbal intelligence $(r = .38, p < .001)$.

Teacher ratings of child verbal intelligence were most related both with mother-infant interaction and stimulation sequence and with promotion to first grade but other scales of curiosity/ creativity, task-orientation, and independence that are included in a factor of academic competence were also correlated with both maternal behavior and with grade promotion. Teacher ratings of the child's social adjustment of considerateness versus hostility and of extraversion versus introversion had low and insignificant correlations with maternal behavior during infancy and with promotion. The relatively unreliable and unstable dimensions of maternal Punitiveness/Irritability had typically low and insignificant correlations with both child academic competence and social adjustment during kindergarten.

The longitudinal analyses of this study found that mother-infant interaction was significantly correlated with mother's cooperativeness with interviewers, disagreement with external locus of control, and self-directing as contrasted to conforming values for children as well as with mother's receptive vocabulary. A similar set of intercorrelated variables from the kindergarten interview included a rating of maternal language skills; agreement with democratic and disagreement with authoritarian childrearing beliefs; reports of providing educational experiences, of talking with child, and of earlier age of teaching academic skills; as well as overall individual modernity scores (Inkeles and Smith, 1974). Significantly intercorrelated measures of individual and parental modernity were summed with equal weights to develop psychosocial environment scores for infancy and for kindergarten data. Both the infancy and kindergarten psychosocial environment scores were substantially correlated with mother's education and with teacher ratings of child verbal intelligence and curiosity/creativity. The intercorrelations among observation and interview data on maternal behavior with child and with interviewer, maternal childrearing beliefs and values, individual modernity, receptive vocabulary, locus of control, and education suggest that each of these measures are indicators of the cultural or psychosocial environment of the child. The psychosocial environment scores had higher correlations than the individual maternal characteristics with teacher ratings of child academic competence. The psychosocial environment scores for white subjects had higher stability (r = .72) from infancy to kindergarten than for black subjects (r = .57). Correlations of the psychosocial environment scores with child verbal intelligence and other competence measures were also higher for white than for black subjects, a finding that is similar to higher predictability of four-year IQ scores for white than for black children in a large sample perinatal collaborative study (Broman, Nichols & Kennedy, 1975).

AN ENVIRONMENTAL INTERPRETATION OF PARENT-CHILD CORRELATIONS

The confounding of genetic and environmental influences upon the development of children reared in their natural families does not allow clear differentiation of those influences. However, evidence for the plausibility of environmental effects includes increases in mental test scores of children during early intervention, decreases after termination of environmental enrichment, and increases in mental test scores of adolescents and young adults after leaving their severely depriving families (Clarke & Clarke, 1976). Evidence of higher IQ scores of children in formerly isolated communities, after improvements in communication and education, also supports an environmental interpretation. Perhaps school desegregation and increased educational, occupational, cultural, and political participation of blacks in the United States subsequent to the civil rights movement have contributed to the narrowing gap between white and black achievement test scores reported by Jones (1984).

Parallel historical increases in mean mental test scores and in educational, technological and scientific development in the United States present even more dramatic evidence of the influence of the cultural environment on intellectual development. Tuddenham (1948) reported substantial increases in mental test scores of United States soldiers from World War I to World War II with the mean of World War II equal to the 82 percentile of World War I. An analysis of changing United States norms on standard mental tests concluded that massive gains have occurred in mean IQ's with an increase of 13.8 points from 1932 to 1978 (Flynn, 1984). Similar increases have been reported in mean IQ in Japan since World War II with a gain of 7 points over a 23-year period (Lynn, 1982).

Bell's (1973) analysis of the post-industrial knowledge society with rapid changes in education, technology, and science may provide an explanation for the apparent increases in intelligence. Etzioni's (1968) parallel analysis of "The Active Society" contrasted man "...as a passive observer in a world not of his making and not under his control" with man as an active self in an active society. Jaynes (1977) monograph on the "Origin of Consciousness..." is similar in an emphasis on a growing awareness of individual autonomy and responsibility during the development of Greek civilization. Feire's (1970) analysis of the culture of silence and of the need for conscientization in an effective "Pedagogy of the Oppressed" emphasizes the need for the development of individual autonomy in low-income, less educated, and oppressed populations. Perhaps parallel increases in knowledge and an active orientation are developed by participation in the educational, cultural, political and economic sectors of society as shown by Kohn's (1969) report that parents in occupations that allow more autonomy have more selfdirecting as contrasted to conforming values for children. Education is substantially related to efficacy, internal locus of control, respect for rights of women and minorities, and democratic as contrasted to authoritarian child-rearing beliefs. Apparently societal development is correlated with individual development of modernity in beliefs, values, skills, motivation, and cognitive functioning. A parent's level of individual and parental modernity influences the child's experience both by provision of educational materials and experiences in the family and community and by parent activities as procurers, advocates, and mediators of societal contributions to child development (Schaefer, 1972). Vygotsky (1978) and Mead (1934) provide detailed analyses of the processes through which shared experiences and verbal interaction of parent and child contribute to cognitive development.

TOWARD AN ENVIRONMENTAL THEORY OF INDIVIDUAL AND SOCIETAL DEVELOPMENT

Integration of findings of significant correlations of parental modernity with child academic competence with historical data on societal development and on increases in mean intelligence of individuals suggests an environmental theory of individual and societal development. Changes in level of individual and societal development through time are indicated in the Figure by a vector from level of development (D1) at time one (T1) to level of development (D2) at time two (T2) for the three domains of societal modernity, individual/parental modernity and child modernity/competence. Vectors connecting each domain with the other domains indicate reciprocal influences, e.g., individual/ parental modernity is influenced by societal modernity and societal modernity is influenced by the individual's active participation and contribution to society. Individual/parental modernity influences the child's modernity/competence as well as the child's subsequent interactions with the parent and the child's participation in society. Similarly society influences child development, with societal influence on child development partially mediated by the parent, and the child's interactions with society partially influenced by the child's level of development. This system of reciprocal influences contributes to the development of the individual parent and child—and to the development of society.

Although longitudinal data suggest that parent influences during infancy contribute to child development, stability of parental modernity over time suggests that parents have a continuing influence on development. Similarly parent and child experiences with education, occupations, and the mass media contribute to their continuing development throughout the life span. The environmental theory of societal and individual development suggests the potential for many different approaches for interventions designed to influence individual development. The theory also suggests that the percent of creative individuals who are capable of making significant contributions to society is not stable or fixed but is increased by investments in human capital (Shultz, 1961) or by progress in societal development.

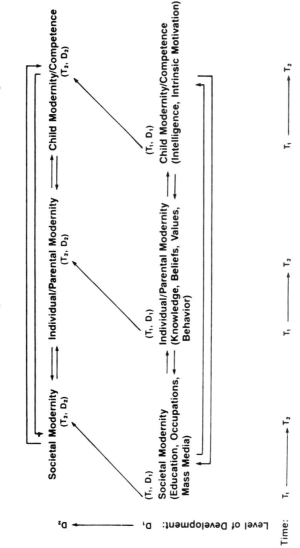

An Environmental Theory of Individual and Societal Development

INDEPENDENCE OF ACHIEVEMENT AND ADJUSTMENT

Societal, adult, and child modernity are substantially correlated with intellectual ability and with educational, and occupational achievement but typically have low and insignificant correlations with social and emotional adjustment of parent and child. Similarly, intimate relationships, that are substantially correlated with social and emotional adjustment, probably have low and insignificant correlations with modern competence of parent and child. Modernity apparently is more highly correlated with cognition than with affect, and with achievement than with happiness and social adjustment. Differentiation of correlates of modern competence from correlates of social adjustment is an important direction for continued research on child development.

IMPLICATIONS FOR RESEARCH

The environmental theory of individual and societal development might contribute to the integration of sociological research on socioeconomic status and psychological research on intelligence by interpreting both as indicators of modern competence of parent or child. Ethnic, racial, or minority group membership might also be interpreted as an indicator of individual modernity that would vary through time as a group is integrated into modern society, e.g., Jones' (1984) data on increases in achievement test scores of blacks.

A fruitful direction for future research is identification and/or development of additional indicators of societal modernity, individual and parental modernity, and child modernity/competence. Inkeles and Smith's (1974) development of twenty scales for different components of individual modernity; the identification of parent beliefs, values, and childrearing and educational behaviors that are components of parental modernity; and the identification of child cognitive and conative variables that are related to child modernity/competence provide a basis for investigation of other correlates of these indicators of modernity. Parent occupation and education and parent and child intelligence are also components of modernity. Findings that beliefs and values as well as knowledge, skills and behaviors are components of individual and parental modernity of adults suggests that similar measures can be identified for children. For example, internal locus of control (Rotter, 1954) is probably an indicator of modern competence for both adults and children. A program of research on components of modernity might investigate additional cognitive orientations— attitudes, beliefs, and values—as well as cognitive skills that are important indicators of modern competence.

IMPLICATIONS FOR SERVICES

The longitudinal research findings and the theory that supports an environmental interpretation of the findings have important implications for early child care and education interventions. Increased understanding of the significance of family and community influences upon child academic competence might contribute to increased investment in the development of human capital (Schultz, 1961). Understanding of the role of active participation by parent and child in the development of individual modern competence might also influence the design and implementation of child care and education services. The identification of parents and children in most need of early interventions might also shift from a focus on biomedical factors to family psychosocial factors that are better predictors of academic competence.

Characteristics of individual and parental modernity that are correlated with child intellectual development may also have relevance for selection and for education of early child care and education personnel. Although each of the characteristics that are indicators of individual parental modernity might be useful, educational and childrearing beliefs and values and observations of teacher behavior with children might complement ability and achievement tests in selection and/or credentialing of teachers. Increased recognition that the modern competence of parents and teachers influences the competence of children might contribute to higher valuation of parenting, child care, and education contributions to individual and societal development.

References

Bell, D. (1973). *The coming of post-industrial society*, New York: Basic Books.
Broman, S., Nichols, P., and Kennedy, W. (1975). *Preschool I.Q.: Prenatal and early development correlates*, New York: Wiley.
Clarke, A.M. and Clarke, A.D.B. (Eds.) (1976). *Early experience: Myth and evidence*, London: Open Books.
Flynn, J.R. (1984). The mean IQ of Americans: Massive gains 1932 to 1978, *Psychological Bulletin*, **95**, 29–51.
Freire, P. (1970). *Pedagogy of the oppressed*. New York: Continuum.
Hunt, J. McV. (1961). *Intelligence and experience*, New York: Ronald Press.
Inkeles, A., and Smith, D.H. (1974). *Becoming modern: Individual change in six developing countries*, Cambridge, MA: Harvard University Press.
Jaynes, J. (1977). *The origin of consciousness in the breakdown of the bicameral mind*, Boston: Houghton Mifflin.
Jones, L.V. (1984). White-black achievement differences: The narrowing gap, *American Psychologist*, **39**, 1207–13.
Kohn, M.L. (1969). *Class and conformity: A study in values*, Homewood, IL: Dorsey Press.
Lynn, R. (1982). IQ in Japan and the United States shows a growing disparity, *Nature*, **297**, 222–23.
Mead, G.H. (1934). *Mind, self, and society*, Chicago: University of Chicago Press.
Rotter, J.B. (1954). *Social learning and clinical psychology*, New York: Prentice-Hall.
Schaefer, E.S. (1961). Converging conceptual models for maternal behavior and for child behavior. In J.C. Glidewell (Ed.), *Parental attitudes and child behavior* (pp. 124–146), Springfield, IL: Charles C. Thomas.
Schaefer, E.S. (1971). Development of hierarchical, configurational models for parent behavior and child behavior. In J.P. Hill (Ed.), *Minnesota Symposia on Child Psychology* (Vol. 5, pp. 130–161), Minneapolis, MN: University of Minnesota Press.
Schaefer, E.S. (1972). Parents as educators: Evidence from cross-sectional, longitudinal, and intervention research, *Young Children*, **27**, 227–39.
Schaefer, E.S. (1981). Development of adaptive behavior: Conceptual models and family correlates. In M.J. Begabb H.C. Haywood, & H.L. Garber (Eds.), *Psychosocial influences on retarded development: Vol. 1. Issues and theories in development*, (pp. 155–78), Baltimore, MD: University Park Press.
Schaefer, E.S., Bell, R.Q., and Bayley, N. (1959). Development of a maternal behavior research instrument, *Journal of Genetic Psychology*, **95**, 83–104.
Schaefer, E.S. & Edgerton, M. (1978). *Classroom Behavior Inventory*. Test Collection, Educational Testing Service, Princeton, N.J. 08541.
Schaefer, E.S. & Edgerton, M. (1985). Parent and child correlates of parental modernity. In I.E. Sigel (Ed), *Parental belief system* (pp. 287–318), New York: Erlbaum.
Schultz, T.W. (1961). Investment in human capital. *American Economic Review*, **51**, 1–17.
Siegel, E., Bauman, K.B., Schaefer, E.S., Saunders, M.M., and Ingram, D.D. (1980). Hospital and home support during infancy: Impact on maternal

attachment child abuse and neglect, and health care utilization, *Pediatrics*, **66,** 183–190.

Simeonson, R.J., Cooper, D.H., and Scheiner, A.P. (1982). A review and analysis of the effectiveness of early intervention programs, *Pediatrics*, **69,** 635–41.

Tuddenham, R.D. (1948). Soldier intelligence in World Wars I and II, *American Psychologist*, **3,** 54–56.

Vygotsky, L.S. (1978). *Mind in society: The development of higher psychological processes* (M. Cole, V. John-Steiner, S. Scribner, & E. Souberman, Eds.), Cambridge, MA: Harvard University Press.

List of contributors

DR. THEO COX

Dr. Theo Cox, Lecturer in Education, University College of Swansea, Wales, England

DR. LEILA BECKWITH

Dr. Leila Beckwith, Department of Pediatrics, School of Medicine University of California at Los Angeles, Los Angeles, CA 90024

DR. SARALE E. COHEN

Dr. Sarale E. Cohen, Department of Pediatrics, School of Medicine, University of California at Los Angeles, Los Angeles, CA 90024

KATHRYN E. BARNARD

Kathryn E. Barnard, Ph.D., Professor of Nursing, Department of Parent & Child Nursing, University of Washington, Seattle, WA

DR. NORMA M. RINGLER

Dr. Norma M. Ringler, Research Consultant, Rainbow Babies & Children's Hospital, University Hospitals of Cleveland, 2074 Abington Road, Cleveland, OH 44106

DR. ROBERT H. BRADLEY

Dr. Robert H. Bradley, Ph.D., Director—Center for Child Development, and Education, College of Education, University of Arkansas at Little Rock, 33rd and University, Little Rock, AR 72204

BETTYE M. CALDWELL

Bettye M. Caldwell, Ph.D., Past President of the National Association, for the Education of Young Children, Donaghey Distinguished Professor of Education, Center for Child Development & Education, College of Education, University of Arkansas at Little Rock, 33rd & University, Little Rock, AR 72204

HUGH LYTTON

Hugh Lytton, Ph.D., Faculty of Education, Department of Educational Psychology, 2500 University Dr., NW, Calgary, Alberta, Canada T2N 1N4

EDWARD E. GOTTS

Edward E. Gotts, Ph.D., Chief Psychologist, Huntington State Hospital, PO Drawer 448, Huntington, West Virginia 25709

DR. EARL S. SCHAEFER

Dr. Earl S. Schaefer, Professor, Department of Maternal, and Child Health, University of North Carolina, School of Public Health 20th, Chapel Hill, NC 27514

AUTHOR INDEX

SUBJECT INDEX